Dana E. King, MD

Faith, Spirituality, and Medicine
Toward the Making of the Healing Practitioner

*Pre-publication
REVIEWS,
COMMENTARIES,
EVALUATIONS . . .*

"**D**r. Dana King has masterly combined his clinical brilliance with a deep appreciation of the beneficial impact of religion and spirituality on the healing of his patients. A timely work of wisdom, insight, and discernment."

Peter Manu, MD, FACP
Professor of Clinical Medicine,
Albert Einstein College of Medicine,
New York

"**T**he opposition between spirituality and medicine has been breaking down, and collaboration is now the word. In his new book, *Faith, Spirituality, and Medicine*, Dana King persuasively shows how medical professionals can actually integrate spirituality in their practice. This is a great addition to any physician's library."

Francis S. MacNutt, PhD
President,
Christian Healing Ministries
Jacksonville, FL

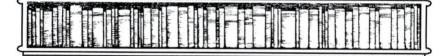

More pre-publication
REVIEWS, COMMENTARIES, EVALUATIONS . . .

"**D**r. King's new work is an important addition to the growing literature on faith and medicine. This book is concise, yet comprehensive. It summarizes a large number of important references published across a wide range of professional literature through 1999, and is meticulously referenced. While it is easy to read in its entirety, it is organized into well-contained chapters that could stand alone. Chapters such as 'Assessing Patients' Spirituality: Taking a Spiritual History' and 'Ethics of Involvement in Patients' Spirituality' could be used independently to impact practice or facilitate discussions among physicians. The text is sprinkled with cases that bring the content alive. Objectives for each chapter and questions for discussion throughout the text make it an excellent resource for classroom use. Overall, this work makes a strong argument for the importance of integrating spirituality into clinical practice and provides practical tools to enable the physician to successfully do so."

Kenneth E. Olive, MD, FACP
Associate Professor
and Interim Chair,
Department of Internal Medicine,
James H. Quillen College of Medicine,
East Tennessee State University

"**A**n impressive body of evidence is revealing profound connections between faith, spirituality, and health. As a result, physicians are no longer justified in standing on the sidelines where these issues are concerned. These developments herald a new era in health care in which meaning and purpose stand alongside biology as vital factors in health outcomes. The result is a form of medicine that works better and feels better, for both patient and physician.

This book is a winner. It is an invaluable aid in introducing health care professionals to the spirituality and health area, and is a reliable guide in applying these findings to clinical practice. *Faith, Spirituality, and Medicine* is free of advocacy and does not evangelize. Its strength is empirical evidence, mixed with compassion and common sense."

Larry Dossey, MD
Author, *Reinventing Medicine* and *Healing Words*

**NOTES FOR PROFESSIONAL LIBRARIANS
AND LIBRARY USERS**

This is an original book title published by The Haworth Pastoral Press®, an imprint of The Haworth Press, Inc. Unless otherwise noted in specific chapters with attribution, materials in this book have not been previously published elsewhere in any format or language.

CONSERVATION AND PRESERVATION NOTES

All books published by The Haworth Press, Inc. and its imprints are printed on certified pH neutral, acid free book grade paper. This paper meets the minimum requirements of American National Standard for Information Sciences–Permanence of Paper for Printed Material, ANSI Z39.48-1984.

Faith, Spirituality, and Medicine
Toward the Making of the Healing Practitioner

THE HAWORTH PASTORAL PRESS
Religion and Mental Health
Harold G. Koenig, MD
Senior Editor

New, Recent, and Forthcoming Titles:

A Gospel for the Mature Years: Finding Fulfillment by Knowing and Using Your Gifts by Harold Koenig, Tracy Lamar, and Betty Lamar

Is Religion Good for Your Health? The Effects of Religion on Physical and Mental Health by Harold G. Koenig

Adventures in Senior Living: Learning How to Make Retirement Meaningful and Enjoyable by J. Lawrence Driskill

Dying, Grieving, Faith, and Family: A Pastoral Care Approach by George W. Bowman

The Pastoral Care of Depression: A Guidebook by Binford W. Gilbert

Understanding Clergy Misconduct in Religious Systems: Scapegoating, Family Secrets, and the Abuse of Power by Candace R. Benyei

What the Dying Teach Us: Lessons on Living by Samuel Lee Oliver

The Pastor's Family: The Challenges of Family Life and Pastoral Responsibilities by Daniel L. Langford

Somebody's Knocking at Your Door: AIDS and the African-American Church by Ronald Jeffrey Weatherford and Carole Boston Weatherford

Grief Education for Caregivers of the Elderly by Junietta Baker McCall

The Obsessive-Compulsive Disorder: Pastoral Care for the Road to Change by Robert M. Collie

The Pastoral Care of Children by David H. Grossoehme

Ways of the Desert: Becoming Holy Through Difficult Times by William F. Kraft

Caring for a Loved One with Alzheimer's Disease: A Christian Perspective by Elizabeth T. Hall

"Martha, Martha": How Christians Worry by Elaine Leong Eng

Spiritual Care for Children Living in Specialized Settings: Breathing Underwater by Michael F. Friesen

Broken Bodies, Healing Hearts: Reflections of a Hospital Chaplain by Gretchen W. TenBrook

Shared Grace: Therapists and Clergy Working Together by Marion Bilich, Susan Bonfiglio, and Steven Carlson

The Pastor's Guide to Psychological Disorders and Treatments by W. Brad Johnson and William W. Johnson

Faith, Spirituality, and Medicine: Toward the Making of the Healing Practitioner by Dana E. King

Faith, Spirituality, and Medicine
Toward the Making of the Healing Practitioner

Dana E. King, MD

The Haworth Pastoral Press®
An Imprint of The Haworth Press, Inc.
New York • London • Oxford

Published by

The Haworth Pastoral Press®, an imprint of The Haworth Press, Inc., 10 Alice Street, Binghamton, NY 13904-1580

© 2000 by The Haworth Press, Inc. All rights reserved. No part of this work may be reproduced or utilized in any form or by any means, electronic or mechanical, including photocopying, microfilm, and recording, or by any information storage and retrieval system, without permission in writing from the publisher. Printed in the United States of America.

Cover design by Jennifer M. Gaska.

Library of Congress Cataloging-in-Publication Data

King, Dana E., 1956-
  Faith, spirituality, and medicine : toward the making of the healing practitioner / Dana E. King.
     p.   cm.
  Includes bibliographical references and index.
  ISBN 0-7890-0724-X (hard : alk. paper)—ISBN 0-7890-1115-8 (soft : alk. paper)
  1. Medicine—Religious aspects. 2. Medical education. I. Title.

BL65.M4 K55 2000
291.1′75—dc21   00-038329

To Kathy, Karen, and Steven

CONTENTS

About the Author   xi

Contributors   xii

Foreword   xiii
    Harold G. Koenig

Acknowledgments   xvii

**Chapter 1. Integrating Religion and Spirituality
into the Biopsychosocial Model**   1
    Dana E. King
    Harold J. May
    Michael E. McCullough
    Dale A. Matthews

    Chapter Objectives   1
    Introduction   1
    The Biopsychosocial Model   2
    Spirituality and Mental Health   5
    Spirituality and Physical Health   5
    A Biopsychospiritual Model   6
    Patients' Desire for Addressing Spiritual Issues
        in the Medical Setting   9
    Spirituality in Practice   9
    Summary   10

Chapter 2. Patients and Religion   13

    Chapter Objectives   13
    Introduction   13
    People in the United States Are Religious   13
    Geography of Religion in the United States   14
    Demographics   15
    Health Beliefs of Selected Religious Groups   16
    Summary   19

Chapter 3. Patients and Spirituality   21

Chapter Objectives   21
Introduction   21
Intrinsic versus Extrinsic Spirituality   22
Spirituality During Illness   22
Faith in Spiritual Healing   24
Spirituality and Health   24
Spirituality and Prayer   26
Spirituality and Meditation   29
Summary   29
Questions for Discussion   29

Chapter 4. Religion, Spirituality, and Health   31

Chapter Objectives   31
Introduction   31
Rationale for Studying Religion/Spirituality and Health   32
Religious Commitment and Mortality   34
Religious Commitment and Physiologic/Immune Factors
    in Health   35
Religious Commitment and Depression   36
Summary   37
Questions for Discussion   37

Chapter 5. Health Professionals and Spirituality   39

Chapter Objectives   39
Introduction   39
Spiritual and Religious Beliefs of Health Professionals   39
The Integration Gap   41
The Spirituality Gap   43
Summary   47
Questions for Discussion   48

Chapter 6. Assessing Patients' Spirituality: Taking a Spiritual History   49

Chapter Objectives   49
Introduction   49
Why Assess Patients' Spirituality?   49

When Should Patients' Spirituality Be Assessed? 54
How to Take a Spiritual History 56
FICA 58
MERIT 61
Summary 62
Questions for Discussion 62

Chapter 7. Ethics of Involvement in Patients' Spirituality 63

Chapter Objectives 63
Introduction 63
Ethics of Spiritual Inquiry 64
Ethics of Referral to Chaplains 66
Ethics of Prayer with Patients 68
Summary 69
Questions for Discussion 69
Cases for Discussion 70

Chapter 8. Chaplains and Pastoral Services 73

Chapter Objectives 73
Introduction 73
Education and Training 73
Role of the Chaplain 76
Collaborating with Chaplains in the Treatment
  of Patients 80
The Impact of Pastoral Care on Health 82
Summary 84
Questions for Discussion 84

**Chapter 9. Spirituality in Special Patient Populations:
Dying Patients 85**

Chapter Objectives 85
Introduction 85
The Role of Spirituality in End-of-Life Decisions 86
Spirituality As a Coping Mechanism 88
Belief in Miracles and an Afterlife 90
Summary 91
Questions for Discussion 91

Chapter 10. Spirituality in Special Patient Populations: Surgical Patients　　　　**93**

Chapter Objectives　　　　93
Introduction　　　　93
Before Surgery　　　　93
Surgery and Prayer　　　　94
Religious/Spiritual Factors and Surgical Recovery　　　　95
Addressing Spiritual Concerns and Mobilizing
　　Spiritual Resources in the Surgical Patient　　　　95
Summary　　　　96
Question for Discussion　　　　98

Chapter 11. Integrating Spirituality into Clinical Practice　　　　**99**

Chapter Objectives　　　　99
Introduction　　　　99
Spectrum of Involvement　　　　100
Integrating Spirituality into Health Professions Education　　　　103
Summary　　　　105

Notes　　　　**107**

Index　　　　**121**

ABOUT THE AUTHOR

Dana E. King, MD, grew up in Ohio and attended Miami University in Oxford, Ohio, where he received a BA in chemistry. He graduated from the University of Kentucky College of Medicine in 1981 and was inducted into AOA, the national medical honorary. He served at the University of Maryland as Co-Chief Resident.

Dr. King is currently Associate Professor of Family Medicine at the Medical University of South Carolina. He has also been Associate Professor of Family Medicine at the East Carolina University School of Medicine, where he developed and directed a required curriculum for medical students regarding faith, spirituality, and medicine.

Dr. King was selected as one of sixty researchers in the field to participate in a national consensus conference in 1996. He has presented his work nationally and internationally and is a persistent advocate for the integration of spirituality into the care of patients.

CONTRIBUTORS

Dale A. Matthews, MD, FACP, practices general internal medicine in Washington, DC, and teaches at Georgetown University School of Medicine. He is the author of *The Faith Factor: Proof of the Healing Power of Prayer,* Viking, 1998.

Harold J. May, PhD, is Professor and Head of Behavior Medicine in the Department of Family Medicine at the East Carolina University Brody School of Medicine, Greenville, North Carolina.

Michael E. McCullough, PhD, is Director of Research at the National Institute for Healthcare Research in Rockville, Maryland. Previously he was Assistant Professor at Louisiana Tech University, Ruston, Louisiana.

Foreword

Research demonstrating a link between traditional religious beliefs and practices and health is rapidly expanding, threatening to bring down the wall of separation between religion and medicine. The teaching and practice of medicine is changing as a result of these findings. In 1992 only about five of the 126 medical schools in the United States had required or elective courses in religion, spirituality, and medicine. Today over sixty such courses exist, including those at major teaching centers such as Harvard, Johns Hopkins, Brown, Case-Western, University of Chicago, University of Pennsylvania, Washington University at St. Louis, and others. Despite this, much controversy remains regarding whether and how doctors should address the religious and spiritual needs of patients.

Articles in prominent medical journals have expressed concerns about the ethical implications of clinicians bringing up religion in the context of a medical evaluation, particularly in the absence of clear guidelines. Will physicians impose their own religious beliefs on vulnerable patients? Will patients' religious and spiritual beliefs be honored, even if different from those of the physician? Will doctors prescribe religious practices such as going to church or praying to nonreligious patients, just as they encourage patients to exercise and stop smoking? Will such prescriptions induce guilt over moral failures if patients refuse such advice and then become ill or fail to recover? Should boundaries be drawn on how far physicians go in addressing these issues? What are those boundaries? Where does the chaplain—the true professional with years of training in this area—fit into the picture? These and many similar questions bewilder and confuse both health and religious professionals, and are likely to concern many patients as well. A critical need exists for education and training guidelines in this area.

Dr. Dana King, a widely known and respected academician, experienced teacher, and compassionate clinician, provides us with a practical, easy-to-read, informative guide for teaching health professionals how to apply to clinical practice the findings from recent research on religion, spirituality, and health. Until now no single resource has been available to help train health professionals to address this deeply sensitive topic. Consequently, the quality of training in medical school and other teaching programs has been highly variable. This long overdue book will go a long way toward standardizing the types of training that clinicians receive, and therefore fills a huge need.

The contents of this volume are outstanding. First, Dr. King provides us with a biopsychosocial-spiritual model that helps place this entire area into perspective, stressing the importance of viewing the patient as a physical, psychological, social, and spiritual being. If clinicians ignore any one of these human aspects, they will miss an opportunity for effective treatment and healing of the whole person. He then carefully examines systematic research to demonstrate the role that religion and spirituality play in the lives of patients, and their relationship to mental and physical health. Taking a spiritual history, exploring the ethics of physicians addressing spiritual needs, and timely use of chaplain services are all systematically and carefully addressed, as is the special role of religion and spirituality in the care of dying patients and those undergoing life-threatening surgery. The impact that spirituality plays in the lives of health professionals themselves is also examined, with an exploration of how this may affect the quality of care that they provide and the fulfillment and satisfaction they experience at work. Clinician spirituality has been highly neglected in clinical research, and yet has a potentially enormous impact on patient care and health outcomes.

Dr. King's volume is the first step toward providing uniform guidelines for training doctors and other health professionals that are necessary for sensitively and comprehensively addressing the religious and spiritual needs of patients. Today, managed care and heavy workloads threaten to drain the joy and satisfaction from the practice of medicine. Bringing the spiritual back into clinical practice provides hope for rectifying this situation and fulfilling the dream of truly helping people, which I believe is the real reason many individuals choose careers in medicine. Treating the whole person is simply *good medicine* for both doctor and patient, and this book will help make it happen.

Harold G. Koenig, MD
Associate Professor of Psychiatry and Medicine,
Director, Center for the Study
of Religion, Spirituality, and Health,
Duke University Medical Center

Acknowledgments

The author wishes to thank Jerri Harris for editorial assistance, and Susan Loftin, Tara Hogue, and Pam Beasley for their typing assistance. Many thanks also to Harold Koenig, MD, David B. Larson, MD, and Dale Matthews, MD, for their inspiration and work in the field.

Chapter 1

Integrating Religion and Spirituality into the Biopsychosocial Model

Dana E. King
Harold J. May
Michael E. McCullough
Dale A. Matthews

CHAPTER OBJECTIVES

1. To review the current biopsychosocial model
2. To review recent empirical literature that supports an association between religion/spirituality and physical/mental health
3. To understand how a biopsychospiritual model better recognizes the influence of religious commitment and spirituality on health
4. To understand the features of an expanded biopsychospiritual model and its usefulness in clinical practice

INTRODUCTION

The biopsychosocial model is a framework for understanding the integration of the biological, psychological, and social dimensions of health and disease.[1] In this model, psychological stressors are recognized as shaping physiologic processes through a variety of neural and hormonal pathways.[2] This influential and widely used model may need to be expanded in view of the growing recognition of the importance of religious and spiritual issues in medical care, and the inability of the current model to explain the effect of religious commitment and spirituality on health beliefs and medical outcomes.[3,4]

Recent research findings support the need to expand the biopsychosocial model to include spirituality. A review of 1,086 studies in the family medicine literature by Craigie, Larson, and Liu has shown a positive association of spirituality on health in 75 percent of the studies that included spiritual variables.[5] Matthews and Larson have published a four-volume annotated bibliography of over 300 studies that link religion and spirituality to health.[6] Levin has reviewed possible mechanisms for these correlations, including social support, physiologic effects of meditation and prayer, psychodynamics of ritual, faith and belief, avoidance of risk, enhancement of healthy lifestyle behaviors, and supernatural effects (effects of God or a Higher Power through unexplained means).[7,8] Such evidence has not led to substantial discussion of spirituality in the biopsychosocial literature; a recent review of eight leading psychology journals found less than 3 percent of quantitative studies included any religious or spiritual variables; only 1.2 percent of psychiatry studies include such variables.[9] The biopsychosocial model cannot be said to include spirituality when so few researchers include it as a factor in their research.

In this chapter, we propose that the biopsychosocial model as currently articulated is inadequate to explain the growing body of evidence supporting the influence of spirituality on health, and that the biopsychosocial model be expanded to include the influence of religion and spirituality to more fully explain health behaviors and outcomes. We will review the basis for the current biopsychosocial model, the body of research reflecting the substantial influence of spirituality on health, and patients' desire for attention to their spirituality in the health care environment.

THE BIOPSYCHOSOCIAL MODEL

The prevailing biopsychosocial model has been developed and refined over the past twenty-five years in response to much research on the influence of psychosocial factors, family support, and stress on the biology of health. The utility of this model initially was supported by research showing general correlations between psychological and medical factors, and subsequently confirmed by intervention studies showing the influence of psychosocial variables on medical outcomes.[8,10-12] What was once a provocative idea has evolved into a widely accepted concept that psychosocial factors, family support, and stress can affect health and illness. The model is well accepted, despite the lack of a unifying biophysiological explanation of the health effects of psychosocial support.

Prior to the advent of the biopsychosocial model, the dominant orientation in medicine was the biomedical model, based on a seventeenth-century scientific worldview (exemplified by Newton and Descartes) characterized by reductionism, mechanistic thinking, and mind-body dualism.[10] Reductionism assumes that the understanding of a complex entity can best be achieved by identifying and analyzing its component parts, from which the whole can be reconstructed. It fosters a view that nature is composed of discrete entities interacting in a linear, causal fashion and encourages the development of mechanistic cause-and-effect relationships to explain medical phenomena. Dualism separates the influences of the mind and body on health and behavior.

Much of the health information about a patient is gathered in the context of an ongoing relationship with the physician; the doctor-patient relationship is built on communication. The biomedical model did not acknowledge the impact of the doctor-patient relationship. In developing these concepts, George Engel proposed that the true meaning of both health and illness can be understood only by recognizing and incorporating the patients' concerns in the context in which they live and work.[13,14]

The biopsychosocial model expanded the biomedical model by focusing attention on a range of psychological, social, and family issues germane to health and illness.

One of the best-known examples of this model is the Type A behavior pattern as initially defined by Friedman and Rosenman.[15] Their investigation contributed to the recognition that this behavioral pattern, characterized by time urgency, perfectionism, and reaction to frustration with hostility, was a primary risk factor in the development of coronary artery disease (CAD). In recent work at the Montreal Heart Institute, researchers found that it is possible to successfully predict which patients would experience a recurrence of health problems twelve months after a myocardial infarction, based on the presence of negative emotions such as depression, anxiety, and anger.[16]

Further support for the biopsychosocial model has come from studying patients' psychological and physiological responses to cancer. Greer, Morris, and Pettingale found that women diagnosed with breast cancer who refuse to lose hope have a better prognosis than those who passively accept their disease.[17] The physiologic response to bereavement was studied by Schleifer and colleagues,[18] who monitored the immune systems of husbands of women with breast cancer. The husbands had a suppression of lymphocyte function within one month following their spouse's death; suppression lasted an average of fourteen months. Finally, Cohen and Rodriquez[19] reported finding that psychological stress not only increased the risk of contracting an infectious disease, but also showed that the greater the stress, the greater the risk.

Research findings supporting the biopsychosocial model allowed researchers to expand the conceptual view to medicine and to re-examine the manner in which medicine is practiced. In developing this model further, McWhinney[20] has suggested that the following issues be incorporated into health care: disease prevention, the patient's environment, communication, and the meaning of the illness for each patient. In addition, he suggested that physicians must integrate the body, mind, and spirit in their approach.

The challenge issued by McWhinney to integrate the body, mind, and spirit invites us to advance this model. Further, psychosocial factors do not fully explain the influence on health of such factors as the impact of faith and belief. Religious commitment has been correlated with enhanced survival, increased quality of life, reductions in alcohol and drug use, lower rates of mental illness, and enhanced recovery from medical and surgical illness.[21-24] Such correlations are not fully explained in terms of psychosocial support and stress management.

The biopsychosocial model does not recognize explicitly the influence of religious commitment and spirituality on health.

A recent study of 2,025 residents of Marin County, California, offers an example of the lower mortality associated with religion and spirituality.[25] In this study, community-dwelling residents ages fifty-five years and older were followed for five years; a variety of factors were tracked to determine associations with mortality. The authors controlled for demographic variables (age, sex, race, ethnicity, income, education, employment), presence of chronic disease, functional status, health habits (smoking, alcohol, exercise, others), social participation, and psychological variables (depression, fearfulness, others). Weekly attendance at religious services was the strongest predictor of lower mortality. The influence of religious attendance went beyond social support in this study: volunteers for the Rotary Club and other community groups did not have significantly lower mortality when considered separately from religious attendance.

SPIRITUALITY AND MENTAL HEALTH

A number of studies demonstrate that religious involvement and spiritual well-being are related to fewer reported symptoms of anxiety, depression, and suicidal ideation.[26-30] The majority of research evidence also demonstrates that religious involvement is an important predictor of life satisfaction and well-being.[31] In addition, over forty studies also show that religious involvement and spirituality are associated with lower rates of substance use.[32,33]

Despite the generally health-promotive effect of religious involvement on mental health variables, some aspects of religious faith are related to worse, not better, mental health outcomes. A belief that God is wrathful and punishing, for example, has been shown to be related to negative mental health outcomes.[34] "Extrinsic" religious commitment, which is characterized as commitment based on factors outside the person such as social gain or external authority, is associated with poorer health. "Intrinsic" religious commitment, characterized by unforced inner commitment for spiritual reasons and internal satisfaction, is associated with more positive mental health.[35]

SPIRITUALITY AND PHYSICAL HEALTH

Patterns of disease and mortality vary across religious groups.[36] At least nine published studies have now examined the relationship between measures of spirituality or religious involvement and hypertension.[37-45] Seven of these nine studies, which included subjects from a variety of ethnic backgrounds, religious backgrounds, and age groups, showed that increased religious involvement was associated with lower blood pressure. Thus, it appears that greater religious involvement (as measured by variables such as frequency of attending worship services, and self-reported strength of one's religious beliefs) is related to physical health. These studies provide a link between self-reported involvement in spirituality or religious pursuits and a measurable physiological marker of physical health, and may offer a partial explanation for the lower mortality seen in epidemiologic studies. Other studies have examined whether religious involvement and spirituality are related to other physiological indices of physical health. One recent study found an association between frequent worship attendance and a measure of immune functioning (interleukin-6),[46] suggesting that spirituality may facilitate physical health by altering the immune response.

Although the associations among indices of mental health, physical health, and mortality need further clarification, the available data demonstrate the relevance of spirituality and religious involvement in understanding physical health and illness.

Greater spirituality and religious commitment are associated with lower blood pressure, less depression and anxiety, and lower overall mortality.

A BIOPSYCHOSPIRITUAL MODEL

An expanded biopsychospiritual model would add the spiritual dimension to the current biopsychosocial model and would include spirituality with God, nature, the inner self, or other beliefs that provide meaning to patients' lives. Features of this expanded model include taking into account patients' beliefs, faith, prayer, and other religious practices. Incorporating the model into medical practice would include taking a spiritual history as a routine part of the complete medical examination. Physicians and other health professionals would assess patients' spiritual needs and refer patients for spiritual counseling when indicated, just as they might refer patients to other consultants for psychological or medical needs. The expanded biopsychospiritual model provides a framework for integrating spirituality into clinical practice, provides a more inclusive model for interpreting research in the field, and invites physicians to consider the spiritual aspects of their patients' lives.

Taking into account patients' spirituality is not "alternative" medicine. It demonstrates sensitivity to an integral part of the whole person, a part that exists independently from considerations of health and illness. Spirituality, often expressed in an organized religious faith, is a context for interpreting life events, unrelated to alternative approaches such as herbs, natural remedies, or chiropractic manipulation. Patients do not "adopt" spirituality as a medical therapy; they bring it with them into the medical encounter as an integral part of their lives.

Research on the use of religion and spirituality as a coping mechanism in medical illness offers support for the biopsychospiritual model. Koenig and colleagues have documented patient use of religion and spirituality as coping mechanisms in anxiety and depression among the elderly.[22,47] Reliance on religion and spirituality as a coping mechanism among the elderly is also supported by epidemiological surveys.[48] Pressman and colleagues[26] investigated religious beliefs, depression, and ambulation status in elderly women with broken hips. They found that patients with stronger religious beliefs and practices were significantly less depressed at the time of hospital discharge, even when controlling for severity of illness. In addition, patients with stronger self-reported religious beliefs had better ambulation status at discharge ($p < .002$). Gorsuch's review[32] of the religious aspects of substance abuse treatment and recovery also illustrates the interaction between religious commitment and a health problem involving complex overlapping influences and psychosocial factors. These studies and others support the development of an expanded biopsychospiritual model.

Evidence correlating religious and spiritual behaviors with improved physical health outcomes also lends support to the expanded model.[25,40,46] One study of obstetric outcomes illustrates the possible influence of spirituality on physical health in one particular population.[21] In this study, 1,919 obstetric patient records were reviewed; the religious affiliation of the mother was compared to the rate of neonatal intensive care unit (NICU) admissions. NICU admissions were significantly lower for religiously affiliated patients than for patients with no religious affiliation. After controlling for psychosocial and medical confounders (age, parity, mental status, payment method, and obstetric risk factors), the association of religious affiliation and lower NICU admission rates remained significant (p = .02).

Researchers have investigated other spiritual factors in an attempt to explain correlations in the biopsychospiritual model. One method has been to focus on the effect of spirituality and "intrinsic religiousness" (i.e., unforced inner expressions of belief in a forgiving, loving God) rather than the more negative extrinsic religious influence (externally forced or authoritative God). A widely used spiritual intervention, the twelve-step program in AA, appears to have a beneficial health effect on the basis of a change in intrinsic religiousness.[49,50] Another spiritual factor which is beginning to be studied is prayer, both "local" hands-on prayer, and "nonlocal" prayer at a distance. Laboratory and clinical investigations have been conducted using prayer in an attempt to influence biological health through heretofore unexplained means, but the results of these studies have been not been replicated by others.[3,51]

One recent controlled study evaluated the effect of distant spiritual healing in a population of forty patients with advanced AIDS.[52] This randomized, double-blind trial used a variety of healers in an attempt to positively influence the course of patients' illness. The intervention occurred remotely from the location of the patients, and included prayer, psychic healing, shamanic traditions, and other forms of meditative healing. After six months, treated subjects had significantly fewer AIDS-defining illnesses, fewer doctor visits, fewer hospitalizations, and improved mood compared to control subjects, despite having no significant differences in CD4 counts.

The expanded biopsychospiritual model provides a framework for integrating spirituality into clinical practice, provides a more inclusive model for interpreting research in the field, and invites physicians to consider the spiritual aspects of their patients' lives.

PATIENTS' DESIRE FOR ADDRESSING SPIRITUAL ISSUES IN THE MEDICAL SETTING

Another reason for using an expanded biopsychospiritual model is that many patients welcome prayer and desire to have their spiritual concerns addressed by physicians. King and Bushwick[53] surveyed inpatients at two hospitals and found that 94 percent of patients agreed that their spiritual health was as important as their physical health, and 77 percent wanted their personal physician to consider their spiritual needs. Forty-eight percent wanted their physician to pray with them. These desires are not being addressed by physicians, since 80 percent said their physicians had never or rarely discussed such issues with them. Maugans and Wadland[54] had similar findings among outpatients in a New England survey; 40 percent of patients wanted prayer or religious issues addressed by their physicians, but most reported that these discussions did not take place. A national poll released by Harvard Medical School supported that patients want their spiritual issues addressed in the medical setting.[55]

Many patients express spiritual needs and a desire for direct involvement of their physicians in spiritual concerns. Indeed, over 75 percent of surgical patients and over 80 percent of psychiatric patients indicate that they have three or more specific religious or spiritual needs during hospitalization.[56] The fact that patients request consideration of these needs is not justification for doing so on its own, but when combined with the scientific evidence reviewed, represents an important synergy. With an expanded biopsychospiritual model, patients do not have to ignore or compartmentalize their spiritual faith, but can be encouraged to utilize it when confronting an illness or injury.

SPIRITUALITY IN PRACTICE

Sufficient data are available to support a revision of the biopsychosocial model initially proposed by Engel. An expansion of this paradigm would allow the inclusion and incorporation of spirituality into routine clinical care, an issue that has clear support from the patient's point of view. The report by McBride and colleagues, using a spiritual assessment instrument (INSPIRIT) offers an example of the types of questions physicians could use to facilitate discussions with patients on spiritual issues.[57] As McBride's report indicates, inclusion of a spiritual history can be both time efficient and effective in clarifying important values concerning health and illness.

Learning to obtain a spiritual history should be integrated into basic undergraduate medical education. Some providers are now advocating inclusion of this type of questioning during routine history and physicals. Others view this aspect of communication as crucial during serious medical illnesses and end-of-life care. Inquiry into patient spirituality may assist the practitioner in being culturally sensitive when presenting treatment options and prioritizing medical issues. Such a caring approach will enhance relationships with patients and improve patient satisfaction and compliance. Medical schools should promote awareness of the importance of patients' spiritual beliefs and teach students to utilize appropriate community and hospital resources such as chaplains, ministers, spiritual leaders, or trained mental health providers for complex spiritual issues.[58,59] Greater understanding of spiritual needs and available resources may assist physicians to encourage coping strategies in the patient's own religious or spiritual tradition.

Patient assessment and management strategies change based on new findings and discoveries. The introduction of the biopsychosocial model represented a major adjustment in medical thought based on studies of the physician-patient relationship, the patient's psychosocial variables, and their effect on health and illness. The biopsychospiritual model is in the early stages of development and further research is required. Just as the biomedical model was challenged by a more integrative biopsychosocial model, the next dimension of medical inquiry likely will add religious and spiritual beliefs to the biomedical, psychological, and social factors that affect health status.

SUMMARY

The biopsychosocial model incorporates biomedical, psychological, and social factors into a clinical approach to patient care. This model is supported by research evidence substantiating the influence of stress, personality type, and social support on medical outcomes. Recent studies documenting the impact of religious commitment on health offer the opportunity to expand the model to include spiritual factors. Researchers have shown that greater spirituality and religious involvement are associated with lower blood pressure, decreased anxiety and depression, and lower mortality. By incorporating patients' spirituality into clinical practice, an expanded biopsychospiritual model would promote closer doctor-patient relationships and better meet patients' needs.

Chapter 2

Patients and Religion

CHAPTER OBJECTIVES

1. To understand the high level of religious commitment in the United States compared with other countries
2. To review the demographics of religious commitment and affiliation
3. To review the health-related beliefs of some representative religious denominations

INTRODUCTION

The rationale for attending to the religious aspects of patients' lives derives from the importance given to it by the patients themselves. Religion is an important part of daily life for 75 percent of the people in the United States and is a prominent influence in society. Religious groups have specific beliefs about health practices and medical decisions that guide the actions of their followers. Knowledge of the major demographic factors and the health views of religious groups is imperative to understanding the influence of religion on patients' lives and health.

PEOPLE IN THE UNITED STATES ARE RELIGIOUS

The Gallup organization has tracked America's religious beliefs for over sixty years, with consistent results over time.[1] Greater participation in worship and interest in religion is found in America than in any other Western nation, including Canada, Europe, the United Kingdom, and Australia. For example, although 95 percent of Americans believe in God, only 88 percent of Canadians, 80 percent of Australians, and 65 percent of Scandinavians do.[2] Fifty-eight percent of Americans believe religion is very important, compared with 36 percent of Canadians, 25 percent of Australians, and only 17 percent of Scandinavians. The same pattern is evident in comparing the United States with non-Western nations. An international Gallup Poll among young adults age eighteen to twenty-nine revealed that 90 percent of Americans believed that religion was very important, but only 38 percent of Japanese and 4 percent of Chinese believed the same. Seventy-six percent of Americans agree that prayer is an important part of their daily life; 61 percent say their faith is the most important influence in their lives.[2,3] Eighty percent believe that the Bible is the actual or inspired word of God.

Americans express their religiousness by associating with a specific denomination (92 percent) and by attending regular worship services (42 percent). In 1997, 87 percent considered themselves Christian (53 percent Protestant, 26 percent Catholic, 8 percent other Christian), while 2 percent were Muslim, 2 percent Jewish, and 2 percent were other religions.[1] These percentages have been stable over the latter half of the twentieth century; the 1957 Census Bureau survey found 66 percent Protestant, 26 percent Catholic, 3.2 percent Jewish, 1.3 percent other religion, and 3.6 percent no religion or religion not reported.[1]

GEOGRAPHY OF RELIGION IN THE UNITED STATES

People in different regions of the United States exhibit differences in their religious denominational preferences. According to Kosmin and Lachman,[4] the United States is divided into four distinct regions according to the dominant denomination: Baptists in the South, Lutherans in the upper Midwest, Roman Catholics in the Northeast, and Mormons in Utah and the other Rocky Mountain States. Baptists are concentrated in Southern states and comprise more than half the residents of Mississippi, Alabama, and Georgia, and almost half of North and South Carolina. In contrast, Catholics constitute a significant percentage in forty-eight of fifty states, but are in proportionately greater numbers in Rhode Island, Connecticut, and Massachusetts.

Lutherans constitute more than a third of the population in Minnesota and North and South Dakota, and nearly a quarter of the population in contiguous states.[4] Mormons (The Church of Jesus Christ of Latter-Day Saints) make up over two-thirds of the population of Utah and are a large part of the population in states around Utah. It is important to note not only the regions in which certain religious groups are more numerous, but their relative absence in other regions of the country. Baptists are found in low numbers outside the South; Mormons are less common outside the West. Americans' religious commitment and spirituality is homogenous in its strength, but heterogeneous and geographically dispersed in its expression.

There are also racial, gender, and age-related trends in religious and spiritual commitment.

DEMOGRAPHICS

Race

Religious commitment is higher among African Americans than whites.[3-4] The Gallup Poll reports that 89 percent of African Americans say that religion is very important in their lives, compared with 59 percent of whites. Eighty percent of African Americans claim church membership, compared with 67 percent of whites; 55 percent attended religious services the previous week, compared with 44 percent of whites. Fifty percent of African Americans are Baptist and 9 percent Methodist; a total of 82 percent are Protestant. Nine percent are Catholic and 1 percent are Muslim; 6 percent claim no religion. Blacks are more likely to be Baptist and Protestant than whites, and less likely to be Catholic.

In contrast to African-Americans, Hispanics identify overwhelmingly with the Roman Catholic Church (67 percent); only 23 percent are Protestant.[4] Religious traditions are less established among Latinos. Only 23 percent of Latino Catholics are currently practicing their faith.

Gender

Women are more likely than men to be church members and express strong religious beliefs.[3-6] The Gallup Poll[1] documents that

72 percent of women claim church membership, compared with 62 percent of men. Seventy percent of women respondents said that religion was very important in their lives, compared to 52 percent of men. Christian religious groups have more female than male members. Female predominance is most evident among Protestant sects. In contrast, non-Christian religious groups show a pattern of male predominance, most notably in Judaism, Islam, and among those who characterize themselves in polls as having no religion.[4]

Age

People maintain strong religious beliefs and identification as they grow older. Except for a small decline among adherents to the Catholic faith, denominational preferences remain stable with increasing age.[4] The increasing median age of members of American mainline Protestant churches has been documented for over a decade;[4] among Presbyterians, Jews, Methodists, and Lutherans, disproportionately fewer are under age twenty-five. In contrast, Baptists and Pentecostals have a higher percentage of members under twenty-five than over seventy-five years of age. The slight decline in the proportion of the older population who are Presbyterians, Jews, Methodists, and Lutherans is not due to switching to other religions with aging, but is due to proportionately less recruiting of younger individuals to those denominations. While denominational preferences vary by age somewhat, overall religious commitment is stable across generations.

HEALTH BELIEFS
OF SELECTED RELIGIOUS GROUPS

People's health beliefs vary according to their culture, education, experience, and other factors. Religious and spiritual beliefs and experiences also shape health beliefs. Many organized religions have specific tenets that affect health, (e.g., Jehovah's Witnesses' proscription against blood transfusions), while other religious beliefs are more general and apply to many medical situations (e.g., "sanctity of life" in Catholicism regarding issues of contraception, abortion, and in vitro fertilization). Individuals' beliefs vary greatly and do not always coincide with the principles of the religious group with which they identify. However, health professionals should be aware of some of the specific health-related beliefs of the major religious groups to promote sensitivity and respect for the moral and religious code that guides the decision making of many patients. The following material is a brief overview of beliefs on medical issues for selected religious traditions. It is intended only as an introduction. Those interested in learning more should consult with local chaplains or clergy.

Catholicism

The Catholic Church is a worldwide church with hundreds of millions of followers. The beliefs of the church are based on the Virgin Birth, Crucifixion, and Resurrection of Jesus Christ. The Pope has final authority on earth over church matters.

Abortion is a grave sin according to the Catholic belief. The essential sinfulness lies in the homicidal intent to kill innocent life.[7] Artificial insemination outside marriage is considered immoral. God's law and authority extend to all life and all things. Euthanasia is also considered immoral; one may not directly cause one's death or the death of another, either through direct action or omission.[7] There are no restrictions on blood transfusions. Contraception and sterilization are unlawful interferences in the Godgiven design of reproduction. Despite the clear teaching of the Catholic Church on moral issues, the overlying Catholic ethic is one of God's love and mercy through Christ, rather than legalism.[8]

Church of Christ—Protestantism

Protestant churches vary in worship style, church organization, and some details of religious ritual, but vary little in health-related beliefs. The viewpoint of the Church of Christ is presented here as a representation of Protestantism because the beliefs are common to most Protestant churches. Beliefs about life and health are derived from the supremacy of God, Jesus Christ as Savior and Lord, and the Bible. Adultery, abortion, and euthanasia would be regarded as unacceptable.[9] The church has no objection to autopsy, contraception, or blood transfusion. Individual medical decisions are made with the guidance of God through prayer, consulting the Bible, and consulting fellow Christians and ministers.

Judaism

Jewish religious heritage dates back 4,000 years to the days of Abraham, as recounted in the Hebrew scriptures. God is one almighty Creator and Lord of all things. Two distinct ideological divisions comprise Jewish tradition, based on the strictness of adherence to Rabbinic law: Orthodox (strict) and liberal/progressive (the law is considered a guideline rather than binding).[10]

Abortion is permissible when the mother's life is threatened, and when the pregnancy is the result of rape. Progressive Jews would also allow abortion in situations of substantial risk of congenital deformity.[10] Autopsies are allowed if certain guidelines are followed. Jewish male children must be circumcised on the eighth day of life unless there is danger to the child's life, in which case it may be delayed.[10] Contraception is permissible. The ethics of Jewish law condemn any deliberate action to hasten death, but guidelines on passive euthanasia are less clear. Jews observe no sacraments or "last rites," but do have an active and complex calendar of holy days and observances throughout the year.[8]

Islam

Islamic moral guidelines are based on the Holy Quran (Koran), which is the supreme scripture from Allah (God) recited by Muhammad the Prophet, and the Hadith, which are the recorded actions and sayings of Muhammad.[8] Abortion after the fetus is formed is considered a crime; an exception may be made if continuation of the pregnancy threatens the life of the mother.[11] Certain forms of contraception are allowed if reasons are valid, but not sterilization. Euthanasia is not permitted. Circumcision is a widely practiced tradition. Blood transfusions are allowed.[11]

Jehovah's Witnesses

Jehovah's Witnesses accept medical and surgical treatment. They follow the Bible; many policies are outlined in the Watch Tower Bible and Tract Society publications. Deliberate abortion would be considered the taking of a human life.[12] Circumcision is allowed and optional. Contraception is allowed unless the method interrupts the development of a fertilized ovum. Active euthanasia is not acceptable, but withdrawing medical support would be allowed when such support is seen as only lengthening the dying process.

Jehovah's Witnesses do not accept blood transfusions based on the sacredness of blood as depicted in the Old Testament Scriptures.[12] They do accept nonblood intravenous fluids such as saline solution, Ringer's solution, and others.

The Society of Friends (Quakers)

Quakers are under no obligation to conform to any particular set of beliefs or code of conduct.[13] They believe that the external spirit exemplified in the life of Jesus should be their guide. They do not proscribe what choices individuals should make regarding abortion, contraception, euthanasia, or other medical issues.

SUMMARY

Most people in the United States express a strong religious commitment to a specific religious denomination. Ninety-five percent of people believe in God. Eighty-seven percent are Christian, with Catholics making up the largest individual denomination (26 percent). The predominant religious denomination varies according to geographic region. Religious affiliation and commitment also vary by race, sex, and age.

Different religious groups hold different views on medical issues such as abortion, euthanasia, and blood transfusions. Review of the medical viewpoints of several religious groups illustrates the variable and sometimes conflicting views held by different denominations. Variation in individuals' interpretation and use of religious

guidelines amplifies the wide range of views that can be encountered in clinical practice. Excellent clinical care requires the clinician to be informed about the medical beliefs of major religious
groups that may guide patients' medical decisions.

Chapter 3

Patients and Spirituality

CHAPTER OBJECTIVES

1. To explain the meaning of spirituality in the medical context
2. To review common expressions of spirituality including faith, prayer, and belief in supernatural healing

INTRODUCTION

Spirituality is a term rich in connotation. For some people it is an expression for an elusive, supernatural concept that cannot be totally grasped. For others it represents another dimension, a world of spirits separate from the world of the five senses. For still others it is a set of concrete beliefs and dogma that represent an ultimate truth that is the basis of everything in this world. For the purposes of this text, the term "spirituality" will be used to mean "a set of beliefs that function to provide meaning to life."[1,2] Spirituality embraces the contrasts of right and wrong, good and evil, sin and forgiveness, as well as the concepts of God and life after death. The underlying assumption of this book is that everyone is "spiritual"; that everyone's life includes the concept of spirituality in some context. In the medical context, people often express their spirituality by the way they make important medical decisions and by the way they view the meaning of illness in their lives. Patients' spirituality often includes their religious commitment (see Chapter 2) but extends beyond formal religious beliefs.

Spirituality includes religion and religious beliefs, but the terms are not synonymous. Religion is a more formal system that provides meaning to life through a common set of beliefs, rituals, and practices. Religion is an important subset of spirituality, and provides the structure for spiritual beliefs for most people.

What is meant by a "spiritual side?" It is commonly held that there are different aspects or contexts for describing people. These include the physical, the psychological, and the spiritual. Each of these contexts has a different vocabulary and point of view, and each provides important insights into people's thought processes, feelings, and behavior. The spiritual context is often described in terms of transcendent thoughts and feelings, in which events are interpreted in a long-term context.

INTRINSIC *versus* EXTRINSIC SPIRITUALITY

Hill and Butler concluded that a discussion of spirituality would be clarified if *intrinsic* factors of spirituality were distinguished from *extrinsic* ones.[3] Intrinsic spirituality is an internally focused belief about God or a higher power that influences life's meaning and provides guidance for living. Extrinsic spirituality is adopted external behavior, which may or may not express spiritual beliefs. For example, individual prayer or Bible study would be considered intrinsic spiritual behavior; church attendance for the purpose of making social contacts would be considered extrinsic. Intrinsic and extrinsic spiritual factors affect health and health behaviors in different ways (see Chapter 4).

SPIRITUALITY DURING ILLNESS

Hospitalization is a situation that can prompt patients to ask spiritual questions and express spiritual concerns (see Photo 3.1). In one study of 200 inpatients in North Carolina and Pennsylvania, 94 percent agreed that spiritual health was as important as physical health.[4] Further, 77 percent of the patients wanted their personal physician to address their spiritual concerns. Almost half wanted their physicians to pray with them. Maugans and Wadland found similar results in a study in New England, in which 40 percent of patients wanted discussion of pertinent religious issues.[5] Among the New England patients, religion was even more important in specific clinical situations such as terminal illness (60 percent), giving birth (48 percent), and major surgery (47 percent). [5]

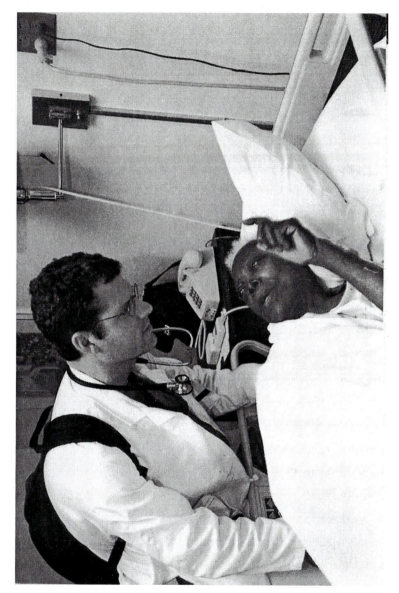

PHOTO 3.1. Patients often express spiritual concerns when hospitalized. Photograph by Margaret Atwood, MUSC Art Services and Digital Imaging. Reprinted with permission of MUSC.

Such results support the idea that patients interpret health and illness in spiritual terms, and do so to a significant extent. The results also support that, as far as patients are concerned, physicians should address their spiritual concerns. Although the desire on the part of patients might be insufficient reason, when combined with evidence that spirituality and religious commitment may affect health (see Chapter 4), such evidence prompts a serious consideration that addressing spiritual concerns should be part of the medical encounter.

FAITH IN SPIRITUAL HEALING

Attention in the media to spirituality and health prompted a national survey, which supports that most patients believe in spiritual healing.[6] Seventy-nine percent of respondents expressed that faith can heal. Over half believed their faith has helped them recover from illness. A regional study examined over 200 outpatients regarding their faith-healing beliefs and found that, while the majority did not believe that faith healers can heal supernaturally, 29 percent believed that faith healers can help some people whom physicians cannot help.[7] Twenty-one percent had attended a faith-healing service, and 6 percent said they believed they had been healed by faith healers.

Faith belief ranges from faith that helps one recover from illness, to faith involving faith healers and specific faith-healing services and rituals (see Case 3.1).* Clinicians should be aware of this "faith spectrum," because not all people who express that they have "faith" are expressing the same meaning. Awareness of the wide diversity of faith belief is especially important for clinicians managing patients facing serious health crises, such as major surgery or end-of-life decisions.[5]

SPIRITUALITY AND HEALTH

Spiritual belief systems have been found to influence coping, recovery, and even specific clinical outcomes.[1,8,9] Measuring spiri-

---

*The unreferenced cases in this book represent real patient situations encountered by the author. Names and some details have been altered to protect the patients' identities.

Case 3.1

Mrs. P. came to the office for her regularly scheduled checkup and to get refills on her medication. She had a history of hypertension and hypothyroidism and had been seen six months previously. Since that time she said she had been doing well. She had no chest pain, headaches, breathing difficulty, or any other symptoms of hypertension. She reported no change in weight, appetite, hair, skin, bowel habits, or other symptoms referable to her thyroid. Her physical examination was unremarkable.

As her physician was refilling her prescriptions, the patient mentioned that she did not need a refill on her thyroid medication. The physician noted that she should have run out of medication by now, and asked her why she didn't need a refill. Mrs. P. was reluctant to answer at first. The physician gently probed further, and she finally admitted that she did not need medicine for her thyroid because she had been "healed." "What do you mean by that?" the physician asked. She explained that she had attended a faith-healing service at her church several months before this visit and had been anointed with oil by the minister. The congregation had prayed for her, laid hands on her, and pronounced blessings upon her. After that experience, she reported that she had faith that she no longer needed the medication and had not taken it in several months.

She still desired a refill of her medication for hypertension. The physician asked about thyroid symptoms again and got the same negative responses as before. The physician asked to check her thyroid stimulating hormone (TSH) level; the patient did not see the need but later agreed. The TSH level returned normal a few days later.

Questions for Discussion

1. What explanation would the patient give for her normal TSH level off of medication? What explanation would you give?
2. How would you react to the story above from a patient of yours? Do you feel it necessary or appropriate for the physician to share a scientific explanation with the patient at his or her next encounter?
3. People who reject standard medical treatment sometimes consider faith healing a last resort or an alternative to traditional Western medicine. How would you explain Mrs. P.'s willingness to continue standard medical treatment for her hypertension, while using faith healing for a different medical ailment?

tual belief has been a challenge for researchers because spiritual belief is a complex set of multiple beliefs, not a simple "level" such as "total cholesterol." The INSPIRIT Index of Core Spiritual Experiences[10] developed by Kass and associates has been used in several studies, and is a tool for measuring intrinsic spirituality. Questions in the INSPIRIT tool explore a variety of inner beliefs. Questions from

INSPIRIT include: How close do you feel to God or a Higher Power? How strongly religious (or spiritually oriented) do you consider yourself to be? Using the INSPIRIT index and a multifactorial instrument to measure health (Dartmouth COOP[11]), McBride and colleagues found a significant correlation between increased spirituality and better patient health (442 patients).[2] This finding supports the hypothesis that health is related to different levels of intrinsic spirituality. Spirituality and health outcomes are discussed in more detail in Chapter 4.

SPIRITUALITY AND PRAYER

Prayer is a common expression of the spirituality of patients. Although some might define prayer as "talking with God," others define prayer more broadly as meditative reflection and communication with a transcendent force or power within or outside the self. Prayer is a prominent part of patients' daily lives, and has been included in research on spirituality and health. Koenig's study showed that prayer is a prominent part of daily activity and coping with illness among the elderly (see Photo 3.2).[12] Maugans' SPIRITual history[1] includes an assessment of personal spirituality and emphasizes the importance of finding out about patients' use of prayer.

Randolph Byrd's randomized clinical trial of the effects of intercessory prayer in a coronary care unit population considered whether specific prayers could affect clinical outcomes.[13] In his study of 393 patients, the prayed-for group had a significantly lower severity of illness during the hospital stay and required less frequent ventilatory assistance, antibiotics, and diuretics than control patients. This study has prompted further investigations and editorials on whether researchers should investigate such a controversial and provocative subject. Based on this study and others some physicians have been prompted to consider integrating prayer into their clinical practice.[14-16] Magaletta and colleagues have proposed a method for introducing prayer into office practice.[17] Others, including Sloan and colleagues,[18] have expressed that empirical evidence and ethical considerations do not support introducing prayer or religious activity into office practice.

Defining an appropriate role for prayer in the medical setting will continue to be a challenge to clinicians. Seventy-five percent of people

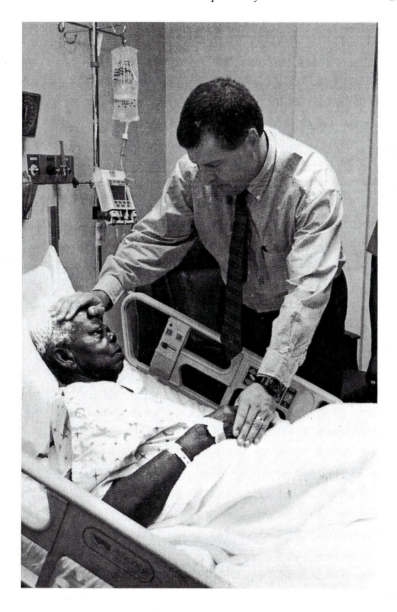

PHOTO 3.2. Patients often use prayer as a way of coping with serious medical illnesses. Photograph by Margaret Atwood, MUSC Art Services and Digital Imaging. Reprinted with permission of MUSC.

consider prayer an important part of their daily lives; the percentage is greater when people become ill enough to be admitted to a hospital. How health professionals address prayer with and for patients has not been well characterized (see Case 3.2). The ethics of prayer with patients is discussed in Chapter 7 and prayer as a coping strategy is discussed in Chapter 9.

Case 3.2

Therapist Judith MacNutt was assigned a new patient, Elizabeth, in the hospital's psychiatric unit. Elizabeth had attempted suicide using alcohol and pills, but had been found and rushed to the emergency department. Elizabeth had been raped by her father and emotionally abandoned by her mother. She had suffered through countless broken, abusive relationships. Her infant son had recently died. Elizabeth felt completely alone, hopeless, and was barely able to speak. She responded to questions with quiet moans, or not at all.

MacNutt counseled her for hours with little progress. She felt overwhelmed by Elizabeth's plight, and turned to God for answers. After praying for Elizabeth and reading Scriptures, she felt a spirit move into her presence like never before. She had a clear vision that she should recruit others to pray for Elizabeth and did so. MacNutt continues the story in her own words:

"Returning to the hospital the following morning after much prayer, I asked to see Elizabeth. She was markedly changed! Her depression had lessened considerably, and she wanted to talk! Although her speech was slow and halting, she began to reveal her innermost fears, disclosing much more than the factual list of traumas she had presented before. She said she felt different and shared something she had experienced the preceding night. She described how she was awakened around 11:00 p.m., precisely when my Christian friends and I were praying. She became aware of a light in her room, although all the lights were out, except for a hall light filtering through her open door. The light (which she recognized as coming from Jesus) enveloped her, spreading warmth and healing love throughout her body and spirit. For the first time in her life, she felt protected and loved. This presence remained with her all through the night, strengthening and ministering to her. Though her outward situation remained unchanged, her heart and deep mind were being healed. As her daily therapy progressed, the walls of pain and isolation slowly eroded. Elizabeth was soon released to outpatient therapy where she continued in her newfound freedom. [*The Healing Line,* Issue 2(3) (Fall), 1998, Christian Healing Ministries, Inc. Permission to reprint granted from Christian Healing Ministries, Inc.]

SPIRITUALITY AND MEDITATION

Meditation is a common practice of relaxation of the body and calming of the mind.[19] Many techniques have been developed, but all have in common a calming and quieting of the body. Spiritual themes of transcendence and finding an inner peace are common to many forms of meditation. Regular meditation has been shown to reduce blood pressure, reduce headaches, and enhance general well-being.[20] Some forms of meditation are derived from the secular context, such as induction of the relaxation response, while others are spiritually based, such as meditative prayers. The beneficial health effects and often spiritual nature of meditation makes this an important aspect of patients' spirituality.

SUMMARY

Spirituality is a set of beliefs that function to provide meaning to life. People express their spirituality in the clinical context through faith, prayer, belief in supernatural healing, and other means. Patients' spirituality influences their view of the meaning of illness and their medical decisions. Clinicians should be aware of the large spectrum of spiritual beliefs in their patients. Later chapters address how to assess patients' spirituality, as well as the ethical questions raised by doing so.

QUESTIONS FOR DISCUSSION

1. What is the difference between intrinsic and extrinsic spirituality?
2. Have you ever had patients express spiritual concerns in the clinical setting? How did you and the medical team respond?
3. How would you respond to a request to pray with a patient?
4. Do you think prayer or meditation will "work better" for psychological conditions than for physical conditions?

Chapter 4

Religion, Spirituality, and Health

CHAPTER OBJECTIVES

1. To explain the rationale for studying the relationship between spirituality and health
2. To review the relationship of religious commitment and mortality
3. To review the effects of religious commitment on physiologic factors, such as blood pressure and immunity
4. To review the use of religion/spirituality in depression and recovery

INTRODUCTION

There is a growing body of literature from clinical and epidemiological studies regarding the association between religious/spiritual factors and physical and mental health.[1-4] The establishment in recent years of the Center for the Study of Religion/Spirituality and Health at Duke University, along with biannual conferences on Spirituality and Healing in Medicine sponsored by Harvard Medical School and the Mind/Body Medical Institute, serve to support the growing interest in the scientific evaluation of religious and spiritual factors. Spirituality can have both positive and negative effects on health. When it provides a sense of meaning, hope, and transcendence, spirituality and religion are associated with better health. When the spirituality or religion is expressed as belief in a punishing and vengeful God, it can have negative effects. Certain sects that avoid medical care from established sources also experience poor health; the mass suicides in Jonestown in 1978 and Heaven's Gate in 1997 are extreme examples of the negative effects of religious cults. The majority of research evidence, however, points to a positive association of spirituality/religion and health.

Craigie and others[2] reviewed 1,086 family practice references to religious factors and health and found that 75 percent of the nonneutral associations were positive. Levin[3] reviewed over 200 studies that showed lower overall mortality or lower rates of specific illness among specific religious denominations. Mathews and colleagues[4] reviewed the empirical literature from over seventy epidemiological and clinical studies relating religious commitment and health status and concluded that religious commitment may play a beneficial role in preventing mental and physical illness. These reviews suggest that although religion and spirituality usually are associated with better health, the association is not universal. Religious commitment varies by age, race, sex, and other factors (see Chapter 2). Such variation underscores the importance of taking a spiritual history from each patient (see Chapter 6) to determine specific beliefs and strength of beliefs.

RATIONALE FOR STUDYING RELIGION/SPIRITUALITY AND HEALTH

Patients presumably do not become religious to gain health benefits, but rather for their own personal and intrinsic reasons. If we cannot "prescribe" religion/spirituality like a drug, why study it? The rationale is based on several factors, all related to the practice of effective health care.

To Learn More About the Patient's Social and Behavioral Context

A patient's social and behavioral context affect health and disease. Just as it is important to learn about patients' marriages and families, it is important to learn about their churches, synagogues, and mosques. Some researchers have suggested that a portion of the benefit of religious commitment and attendance at services is attributable to the social support obtained in a religious congregation.[1,3] Religious affiliation also affects personal health habits—many religious traditions restrict use of alcohol and tobacco, for example.

To Learn About an Important Coping Mechanism

Many people rely on spiritual/religious faith when crises strike, particularly in times of serious medical illness. Religion as a coping mechanism has been shown to reduce depression in elderly hospitalized men, reduce anxiety, and assist in recovery from many types of mental illness and other conditions.[4-7] Hospitalized patients pray for health more than outpatients who are less ill.[8,9] Dying patients are especially prone to rely on faith and spiritual resources, and appear to have less pain and anxiety as a result (see Chapter 9). The aphorism "There are no atheists in foxholes," expresses a common cultural notion of turning to God in times of serious crises. This notion is supported by studies that found that patients who use religious means as a coping strategy seem to cope more effectively than those who do not.[10,11]

To Be Aware of the Variation in Patients' Beliefs

Although two-thirds of people in the United States consider themselves very religious, and 40 percent attend religious services regularly (see Chapter 2), there is a wide range of expression of these beliefs. Most people in the United States are Christian, but many faiths are represented in significant numbers, including Judaism, Islam, and others. The large number of Protestant (Christian) denominations has resulted in a "melting pot" of religious affiliation in the United States, which includes many "independent" congregations that do not associate with any regional or national religious group; members of these congregations often have a variety of unique beliefs and practices. Knowledge of the variation in health beliefs among different religious groups will assist clinicians in asking appropriate questions of patients. Health care professionals would be remiss in assuming religious and spiritual values based on sex, race, or region of the country. Further, there are correlations with various health outcomes among particular religious groups.[3,4]

To Encourage Patients to Use Their Religious/Spiritual Resources for Health Promotion

Matthews and colleagues[4] in their review of religious commitment and health status present several studies to support that religious commitment helps prevent depression, substance abuse, and physical illness, in addition to providing coping strategies and assistance in recovering from illness. These authors suggest that clinicians ask patients how they can support the patient's faith and religious commitment, particularly by promoting the patients' use of meditation, prayer, and other private religious activity. Matthews also suggests referring patients to clergy or chaplains in addition to standard medical care. No current empirical studies show that physicians intervening to promote religious activity among religious patients promote better health. Other authors have cautioned against promoting religion for health's sake, because of concern about imposing one's views on patients, and because "adopting" religion for a health benefit has not been shown to be helpful.

RELIGIOUS COMMITMENT AND MORTALITY

A growing number of studies suggest that religious involvement has positive effects on health and mortality.[12-17] These studies have shown an association of higher frequency of attendance at religious services or other religious involvement with decreased depression, decreased anxiety, improved general well-being, and lower mortality. However, many of the studies had flaws in methodology, including cross-sectional design and exclusion of important confounding factors. Recently, Oman and Reed[13] published a five-year longitudinal study of 2,025 community-dwelling elderly that addressed many of the shortcomings of previous studies. By using all-cause mortality as the main outcome variable, they avoided the reporting biases inherent in intermediate outcomes such as depression or general well-being. By taking into account demographics, health status, physical functioning, health habits, social support, and psychological confounders, they overcame an important problem of previous studies. Although the study still has limitations, including using a predominately affluent white population, its findings warrant review and consideration.

Oman and Reed's[13] study found that weekly attenders of religious services had a significantly ($p < .01$) lower mortality over the average five-year follow-up period than nonattendees, 31 percent lower in men and 34 percent lower in women. This effect was not attenuated among respondents with higher levels of social support. Religious attendance was the only variable among those tested, which showed an independent protective effect against mortality. These findings are consistent with several previous studies showing a protective effect of religious attendance and mortality.[14-16] Whether the attendance at religious services reflects intrinsic or extrinsic religious commitment is unclear.

RELIGIOUS COMMITMENT AND PHYSIOLOGIC/IMMUNE FACTORS IN HEALTH

Hypertension has been the subject of at least nine published studies relating physiologic variables and religious or spiritual commitment.[19-27] Increased religious involvement was associated with lower blood pressure in seven of the nine studies, which involved subjects from a number of ethnic and religious backgrounds. Religious involvement was measured in several ways, including frequency of attending religious services, and self-rated strength of religious beliefs. Levin and Vanderpool[28] reviewed eleven other studies investigating blood pressure differences among different religious groups and found significant differences in all but one study. The finding of lower blood pressure with greater religious involvement implies that the epidemiologic benefit seen in Oman and Reed's study[13] (as well as other epidemiology studies) may be partially explained by physiologic effects of religion on hypertension. A further implication for clinicians is that religious and spiritual factors cannot be considered as having only psychological effects, since religious and spiritual commitment is associated with reduced hypertension, a physiologic effect.

Immune function has also been investigated as a possible factor in the relationship of religion/spirituality and health. Koenig and colleagues[29] followed 1,718 people for three years (ages sixty-five or over) regarding religious service attendance and several immune regulators including interleukin-6 (IL-6). IL-6 is an inflammatory cytokine associated with aging, cancer, heart disease, and psychological stress. Religious attendance was inversely related to high IL-6 levels (greater than 5pg/ml), but not to IL-6 levels as a continuous variable. Religious attendees were only 58 percent as likely (OR [odds ratio] 0.58, 95 percent CI [confidence interval] 0.40-0.84, < .05) as nonattendees to have IL-6 levels greater than 5. The relationship between religious attendance and IL-6 in this study was not attenuated by taking into account depression or negative life events. Many covariates were not considered, and the analysis was not corrected for doing multiple comparisons. Nevertheless, this exploratory study proposes a new area of investigation for possible mechanisms into the association of religious commitment and health.

RELIGIOUS COMMITMENT AND DEPRESSION

Depression affects over 17 million Americans each year, with substantial consequences to patients and families.[30] Effective treatment involves multiple modalities including counseling and medication. Research on the role of spiritual factors in mental illness has focused on depression and has shown that increased reliance on religious coping is associated with fewer depressive symptoms in medical patients. Koenig and colleagues[5] evaluated 850 patients with a variety of medical diagnoses and found that strong personal belief, faith in God, and a relationship with a local congregation was associated with less depression. Another study prospectively evaluated eighty-seven patients with moderate to severe depression over a one-year period.[31] Patients underwent personal interviews, diagnostic tests for depression, and assessment of intrinsic religiousness. The questions on religion focused on inner personal beliefs and the importance of God as a guiding force in patients' lives. After controlling for twenty-eight medical, psychological, and social confounders, intrinsic religiousness was a significant predictor of recovery from depression; church attendance was not. Such data supports that intrinsic (rather than extrinsic) religious commitment is positively related to better mental health.

Religious factors also play a role in the treatment of depression. In a study of fifty-nine patients, Propst and colleagues[32] investigated whether religious patients with depression respond better to cognitive-behavior therapy with or without religious content. Patients receiving therapy with religious content had significantly lower depression scores after treatment than those who received nonreligious therapy. Two other studies using rational-emotive therapy with religious patients did not demonstrate any differences in outcomes between religious and nonreligious approaches.[33,34] Therapy that includes a religious orientation is equal to and sometimes superior to secular-oriented treatment. Further research is necessary to delineate what types of religious content are most helpful in treatment.

SUMMARY

The association of religious and spiritual commitment with better health and lower mortality is important in understanding a patient's social and behavioral context. Patients who use religious means as a coping strategy appear to cope more effectively than those who do not. Several epidemiologic studies have substantiated that attendance at religious services is associated with lower overall mortality. Intrinsic religiousness is associated with more rapid recovery from depression. Therapy that acknowledges the patients' religious background may be superior to nonreligious therapy for religious patients. Clinicians should consider spiritual and religious factors when addressing patients' physical and mental health needs.

QUESTIONS FOR DISCUSSION

1. What do you see as the rationale for studying the association of religious and spiritual factors with health?
2. In what situations have you seen patients using religiousness/spirituality to cope? Was the use of spiritual coping effective?
3. How can knowledge of the effect of religious and spiritual factors on health contribute to an understanding of the medical needs of patients?

Chapter 5

Health Professionals and Spirituality

CHAPTER OBJECTIVES

1. To review the prevalent religious and spiritual beliefs of health professionals
2. To review the beliefs and experiences of health professionals in regard to addressing patients' spiritual beliefs
3. To consider possible effects of health professionals' beliefs on clinical practice

INTRODUCTION

At some point in learning about the spirituality of patients, we begin to look at ourselves and our own spirituality as health professionals. What are our religious and spiritual beliefs? How do they affect our relationships with patients?

SPIRITUAL AND RELIGIOUS BELIEFS OF HEALTH PROFESSIONALS

Physicians, nurses, and mental health professionals have been asked in regional and national studies about their beliefs.[1] In one study of the religious views of marriage and family therapists,[2] therapists were found to have the highest rates of religiosity of any health professional group, especially compared to psychologists and psychiatrists. Fifty percent of marriage and family therapists

39

attend religious services weekly, compared with 43 percent of the general public[3] and less than 27 percent of psychologists.[4] Fifty-five percent of licensed professional counselors and 41 percent of clinical social workers have a current religious affiliation, compared to 67 percent of the general public.[5] Marriage and family therapists may be more likely to be willing to meet patients' religious and spiritual needs since they are more religious themselves. Patients want to have their spiritual concerns addressed when they are ill,[6] and 66 percent prefer a professional counselor who is religious.[7] In light of these studies and others, marriage and family therapy programs are beginning to discuss how to deal with religious and spiritual considerations in their training.[8] Nurses also have a higher rate of religious attendance and affiliation than the general public.[1] Nursing organizations have recognized the relevance of spirituality to their patients; "spiritual distress" has been an official nursing diagnosis since 1988 (North American Nursing Diagnosis Association, 1992).

Family physicians' beliefs and attitudes have been evaluated in both regional and national studies. Maugans and Wadland[9] studied family physicians in Vermont and found them to be less religious than their patients. Beliefs were assessed in a survey, using five different items: existence of God, feeling close to God, God as a personal entity, prayer, and the existence of an afterlife. Only 43 percent of physicians reported they felt close to God, compared with 74 percent of patients. Eleven percent of physicians did not believe in God, compared with national Gallup survey results of 5 percent (see Chapter 2) of the general population not believing in God.

Considerable regional variations are found in the spiritual beliefs of health professionals. Oyama and Koenig[10] studied family physicians in North Carolina and Texas and found rates of church attendance comparable to those of patients in a national Gallup survey. Frequency of other activities were similar to national religious rates, including frequency of use of prayer, meditation, and Bible reading.

Daaleman and Frey's[11] national survey of family physicians showed frequency of religious attendance comparable to the general population as reported in a national survey (73 percent versus 63 percent).[12] The percentage of physicians who felt at least somewhat close to God was 77 percent, versus 84 percent for the general population. The researchers concluded that family physicians' religiousness is comparable to that of the general population. They acknowledged regional variations but were unable to analyze their data by region.

Other health professionals do not have religious beliefs comparable to the general population. Only 43 percent of psychologists and a similar percentage of psychiatrists believe in God, compared to 95 percent of the general public.[4,13] Twenty-seven percent of psychologists attend religious services at least twice a month. This percentage contrasts with the 43 percent of the general public who attend church weekly or more often.[3] In addition, only 33 percent of psychologists agree that "my whole approach to life is based on my religion," compared with 61 percent of the general population.

Although it is clear that significant differences exist among members of different health professions regarding religious and spiritual beliefs, it is less clear how these differences affect relationships with patients. Further research regarding health professionals' spiritual and religious beliefs would be helpful in illuminating the differences between the professional groups and the general population. The next section reviews the manner in which health professionals address spiritual issues with patients.

The spiritual and religious beliefs of health professionals vary by specialty and by region of the country. Nurses, marriage and family therapists, and family physicians have rates of church attendance and religious affiliations comparable to the general public, while psychologists and psychiatrists are less religious.

THE INTEGRATION GAP

Many health professionals struggle with knowing how and when to incorporate spiritual issues into clinical care. Many neglect spiritual issues due to concerns about imposing their beliefs on patients or revealing too much about their own beliefs. At the same time, patients express a strong desire for physicians to consider their spiritual needs.[6,9] To address this "integration gap," Ellis and colleagues[14] studied 231 family physicians in Missouri using the Ellison Spiritual Well-Being Scale and supplemental questions about barriers to addressing spirituality. Ninety-six percent agreed or strongly agreed that spiritual well-being is an important component of good health. Despite this belief, less than 20 percent of physicians discussed any of seven spiritual topics in more than ten percent of patient encounters. However, one-third discussed the topic of fear of death or dying with hospitalized or nursing home patients. Only 22 percent reported using referral to chaplains or other spiritual leaders in more than ten percent of encounters.

Maugans and Wadland[9] surveyed both physicians and patients in Vermont, and found that 77 percent of physicians inquired about religious issues occasionally, and 11 percent frequently or more often. However, the majority of patients could not recall any inquiries by physicians about religious issues. The highest percentages recalled by patients were related to major events such as death (19 percent), major surgery (10 percent), or terminal illness (6 percent). Forty percent of patients responded that they would like physicians to discuss pertinent religious issues.

Olive[15] has looked in more detail into the spiritual experiences and methods of forty self-described devout physicians and found considerable spiritual involvement. This study used twelve interviews and twenty-eight self-administered questionnaires to characterize how these physicians interact with patients. Sixty-seven percent of the physicians had prayed out loud with patients on at least one occasion and they had prayed for patients even more often. Half the time prayer was initiated by the patient, but the physician initiated the prayer equally as often. The physicians discussed patients' beliefs and offered prayer more often in clinical situations involving life-threatening illness and more often if the physician were Protestant. King and colleagues[16] surveyed 594 physicians in seven states across the nation. They found that physicians usually did not discuss religious issues with their patients; 83 percent did so only sometimes or rarely. However, 93 percent of the physicians surveyed agreed or strongly agreed that physicians should consider patients' spiritual needs. This finding is consistent with Ellis's[14] data that 96 percent of physicians felt that spiritual well-being is an important component of good health. Most (61 percent) of the physicians in the King study did not feel that discussing religion would turn away patients from their practices.

Another study[6] reported on a survey of 200 inpatients at two hospitals; one in Pennsylvannia and one in North Carolina; 77 percent said that physicians should consider patients' spiritual needs, and 37 percent wanted their physicians to discuss patients' religious beliefs more. In further defining the desired physician role, 48 percent said they would like their physician to pray with them, and 42 percent expressed that physicians should ask about faith-healing experiences (see Photo 5.1). However, 68 percent reported that their physician had never discussed religious beliefs with them, and 12 percent said they had done so only rarely.

Although both patients and physicians agree that spiritual well-being is important, they usually do not discuss spiritual well-being in clinical situations.

The previous studies illustrate the "integration gap" between the importance of spiritual issues and the relative lack of discussion of those issues. Ellis and colleagues[14] propose several possible explanations: lack of time to discuss spiritual and religious issues; lack of training in obtaining a spiritual history; difficulty identifying patients who want to discuss spiritual issues; and concern about projecting beliefs onto patients. Addressing these issues will be important to improving the quality of care for patients.

THE SPIRITUALITY GAP

The "spirituality gap" is the difference between the spirituality of patients and the spirituality of health professionals. The fact that psychologists and psychiatrists are less religious than most patients means that patients with mental illness will often be treated by someone less religious than themselves.[4,5] How clinicians should approach spiritual differences and how such differences may affect the doctor/patient relationship are not fully known. Although individual variation in type and strength of beliefs inherently raises the possibility of incongruity of beliefs between clinicians and patients, group variation adds an additional dimension for consideration. The

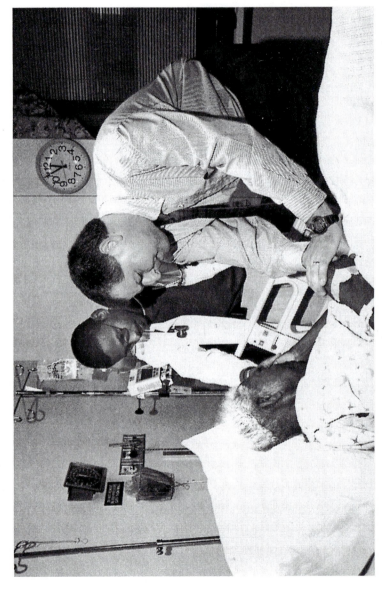

PHOTO 5.1. Some patients would like their physician to pray with them and ask more about spiritual experiences. Photograph by Margaret Atwood, MUSC Art Services and Digital Imaging. Reprinted with permission of MUSC.

large differences in self-professed spirituality between patients and psychologists/psychiatrists are one example of group variation that may affect clinical practice.

A "spirituality gap" exists between patients and health professionals, with patients being more religious and more concerned with religious and spiritual issues than many health professionals, especially psychiatrists and psychologists.

Incongruous spiritual beliefs may affect clinical practice in several ways.

Patient Satisfaction

Since 1996, psychiatry programs have required training dealing with patients' religious concerns (AMA, 1996). Although psychology training programs do not have similar requirements some psychologists have advocated on behalf of such training.[17] The desire on the part of patients to have their spiritual concerns addressed and their preference for a professional counselor who is religious portend deficits in patient satisfaction with current encounters with nonreligious professionals.[6,9,18] The desire for a religious counselor may explain why every year millions of patients seek counseling directly from clergy. Approximately four of ten patients with mental health disorders seek counseling from clergy, which is equal to or greater than the number who seek counseling from psychologists and psychiatrists.[18]

Collaboration in Care

Neeleman and King's[19] study of psychiatrists in London found a wide variation of opinions about the influence of religion on mental health and very few referrals to area clergy. Little collaboration with clergy may reflect negative rather than neutral attitudes about religion and spirituality. While Neeleman and King speculated that many psychiatrists view religion as "peripheral," others have expressed more negative views about religion and health. Watters has written that "Christian doctrine and teachings, deeply ingrained as they are in Western society, are incompatible with the development and maintenance of sound health, and not only mental health, in human beings."[20] He contends that religion is not irrelevant, but actually harmful to patients, and advocates viewing religious conviction as pathology. Viewing religion as harmful does not reflect recent research (see Chapter 4) nor does it allow for collaboration between physicians and clergy.

Variation in Medical Recommendations

Religious and spiritual views of health professionals may affect treatment recommendations. Galanter and colleagues have written on the impact of evangelical belief on religious practice.[21] They surveyed 260 members of the Christian Medical and Dental Society to ascertain how their religious views might affect patient treatment. The respondents considered psychotropic medications most effective for schizophrenia and mania, but would advocate prayer and reading the Bible for alcoholism, grief, and other disorders. One-third of respondents said they would counsel against abortion, homosexual acts, and premarital sex even for nonreligious patients. The American Psychiatric Association has recognized the potential for conflicts between psychiatrists and patients with differing religious views and issued guidelines in 1990.[22]

Quality of Care

The inclusion of religious content in treatment has resulted in improved clinical outcomes for some patients. Propst and colleagues studied fifty-nine patients with depression and found that patients whose treatment included religious content improved more than those who had no religious content in treatment.[23] In another study, daily chaplain intervention in the lives of hospitalized orthopedic patients reduced length of stay and reduced the need for pain medications.[24] More studies are needed to investigate whether including religious and spiritual content as part of treatment is beneficial in other clinical situations.

The spirituality gap may affect clinical practice in several ways, including patient satisfaction, collaboration in care, variation in medical recommendations, and quality of care.

Research has demonstrated that more religious physicians address spiritual issues more frequently than less religious ones. Maugans and Wadland's study showed that physicians who spend two hours a week or more in formal religious activity were more likely to make spiritual inquiries of their patients.[9] King and colleagues found that physicians who had strong religious beliefs were significantly more likely to discuss patients' religious beliefs and ask about faith-healing experiences.[16] If patient satisfaction and quality of care are influenced by recognizing and including religiousness in the treatment of patients, then religious physicians currently may be better equipped to deliver spiritually sensitive clinical care. The challenge is to equip all providers, regardless of their own beliefs, with the skills needed to appropriately assess and refer patients to providers who are sensitive to patients' spiritual needs.

SUMMARY

The spiritual and religious beliefs of health professionals vary by specialty and by region of the country. Although both patients and physicians agree that spiritual well-being is important, they infrequently discuss spiritual well-being in clinical situations. Patients are more religious than many health professionals, especially psychologists and psychiatrists.

Health professionals' religious views affect clinical practice in many ways: some advocate religious views, some view religion as harmful, and some view it as irrelevant. Patients can expect different approaches to treatment from different health professionals. Many patients prefer counselors who are religious, and seek counseling from clergy to ensure that their counselor shares their religious views. Seeking the proper balance of being sensitive to patients' beliefs without imposing one's own is an important issue for all health professionals, and will be examined in Chapter 7, "Ethics of Involvement in Patients' Spirituality."

QUESTIONS FOR DISCUSSION

1. In which specialties are health professionals most religious? Least religious?
2. If health professionals believe that spiritual well-being is important, why do they not discuss spiritual matters with their patients?
3. Describe the "spirituality gap"; the "integration gap." What are the implications of these phenomena for clinical practice?

Chapter 6

Assessing Patients' Spirituality: Taking a Spiritual History

CHAPTER OBJECTIVES

1. To review reasons for assessing patients' spirituality
2. To explore when patient's spirituality should be assessed
3. To review how to assess patient's spirituality and take a spiritual history

INTRODUCTION

Sensitivity to patients' spiritual beliefs and concerns is one of the basic tenets of the biopsychospiritual model. Knowledge about patients' religious beliefs and practices is important for understanding their interpretation of serious illness and desire for treatment. Taking into account patients' religious and spiritual beliefs must include taking a history of their specific religious beliefs and practices as well as an assessment of their spiritual needs and concerns. Patients often rely on their spiritual beliefs as a coping mechanism in times of crises, including major illnesses; the stress of illness may cause a need for more spiritual support and counseling. Sensitivity to patients' spirituality is a clinical skill that can be acquired. This chapter will explore the reasons why it is important to include assessment of patients' spirituality as part of the medical history, when to include such assessment, and how to obtain a spiritual history.

WHY ASSESS PATIENTS' SPIRITUALITY?

Patients' spirituality should be assessed for several reasons, one of which is that over 95 percent of people in the United States believe in God and 80 percent believe that the Bible is the word of God.[1] Just as it is important to determine a patient's psychosocial support, the outline of the family structure, whether a patient is married or has children, and the patient's occupation, it is important to determine the patient's spirituality. Assessment would include the patients' source of spiritual support, general view of his or her context in the universe, and adherence to specific faith traditions. Sixty-one percent of patients profess that their religion is the most important controlling influence in their lives.[2] Because religion and spiritual beliefs are of such importance to a majority of patients, clinicians need to determine their spiritual beliefs about health. A patient's specific religious denomination is also important because it often shapes views about the end of life, blood transfusions, contraception, and other health issues (see Chapter 2).

Other religious beliefs intersect with health beliefs and may influence care. A population survey of 1,052 people in North Carolina found that nearly 90 percent of people believe in healing miracles.[3] Over half of people in one study of 200 patients reported they had experienced or been aware of healing miracles.[4] Seventy-seven percent of inpatients in the same study said that God's will was the most important factor in getting well from an illness, more important than willpower, the doctor's care, or other factors. Such beliefs may have important implications for addressing end-of-life issues, compliance with therapy, and expectations of recovery in the face of serious medical conditions. Research data support the idea that patients are religious and have spiritual lives that are important to them in the medical setting (see Photo 6.1).

Surveys of community and national populations have determined that patients would like to have their spiritual needs addressed (see Chapters 2 and 3). A national study of 1,000 U.S. adults[5] supported that many patients want direct involvement of their physicians in their spiritual health. Sixty-three percent of respondents reported they believe that it is good for doctors to talk to their patients about spiritual faith. Seventy-nine percent believe that spiritual faith can heal and 56 percent said that their faith had helped them recover from illness, injury, or disease. Among specific populations, a higher percentage of patients want their religious and spiritual needs to be addressed during hospitalization. One study documented that 75 percent of surgical

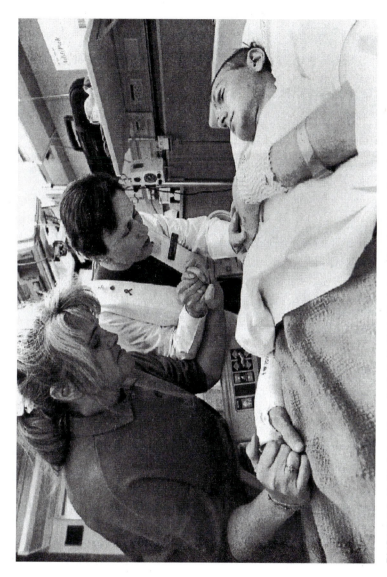

PHOTO 6.1. Patients' religious faith, belief in miracles, and reliance on God's will are often magnified in the medical setting. Photograph Courtesy of East Carolina University Health Sciences Division, News and Information Service.

patients and 80 percent of psychiatric patients had three or more specific religious or spiritual needs they would like addressed.[6]

Thus, the patient's desire is an important reason to assess spirituality, religious health beliefs, and specific spiritual needs. The more serious the medical condition, the more important the assessment for both patient and provider. Mansfield and colleagues have documented an increased reliance on prayer and religious faith among patients who perceived a decline in their health status.[3] Further, surveys of hospitalized patients consistently show higher rates of religious commitment and greater patient need for spiritual concerns to be addressed than patients in outpatient or community settings.[4,6,7] Consequently, inpatients may have a greater need for assessment of their spirituality than outpatients.

Patients' spirituality also should be assessed because of its importance as a source of strength and use as a coping strategy by many patients (see Chapter 9). A growing body of literature on the subject documents prevalent use of spirituality and religious faith as a coping mechanism.[7-9]

Koenig and colleagues' study[10] identified twenty-one different religious coping strategies in a study of 577 medical inpatients. The majority of patients used one or more of sixteen "positive" religious coping strategies, which included collaborating with God, seeking a connection with God, and giving religious help to others. These sixteen types of coping were associated with less depression and better health. Fewer patients used one of the five other religious coping strategies that were associated with poorer health, such as viewing God as punishing or viewing the situation as involving demonic forces. The study reinforces the importance of assessing each patient's spirituality, because patients use their religion to cope in different ways that affect health (see Case 6.1).

Patients' spirituality should be assessed for several reasons:

  1. Patients are religious and have spiritual views that affect health.
  2. Many patients want to have their spiritual needs addressed in the medical setting.
  3. Patients use religious coping in different ways when facing serious illness.

Case 6.1

A middle-aged man began having headaches and mild left-sided weakness and presented to his physician. His physician noted a mild objective left-sided weakness and nystagmus and ordered a computed tomography (CT) scan of the head. The scan confirmed a mass in the right temporal region and the patient was referred to a neurosurgeon. The mass was a malignant brain tumor, the prognosis for survival was approximately six months. The patient and his family were devastated by the diagnosis. The patient and his wife and family were devout Christians, attended church once a week or more often, were active in their Sunday school, and identified their Sunday school class and the church choir as their strongest support groups. The support of close friends and family was also important.

The patient's initial response to surgery and then radiation therapy were profound. He recovered quickly from surgery, returned to his busy insurance practice and returned to his church activities within a month after having brain surgery. He called upon his community of faith and particularly his Sunday school and church choir to pray for him. He and his wife reported that these prayers were earnest and frequent. His condition was frequently reported to the church by means of newsletters and word of mouth. The patient, his wife, and son frequently received donations of food brought to his home without making any specific request. If the patient had any specific physical, transportation, or other needs, he called on his church community for these items and they were almost always provided.

The patient suffered a setback three months later with return of the tumor and faced repeat surgery. He again called on his church community both for social support and for prayer. At the time of the second surgery, the recurrent mass was found to be necrotic tissue and not a recurrence of the tumor. He survived the surgery, made a quick recovery, and returned to work. The patient and his wife attributed this to prayer, a healing miracle, and their faith in God. Eight months after his diagnosis the patient continued to be active, working part-time, and singing in the choir at his church. He attributed his outlasting the doctor's prognosis to God, faith, and prayer.

Questions for Discussion:

1. What evidence is there that the patient's spiritual life was important to him?
2. Would you characterize the patient's use of religious coping as positive, negative, or neutral?
3. Is it relevant to the doctors treating this patient that he has an active religious life?

WHEN SHOULD PATIENTS' SPIRITUALITY
BE ASSESSED?

Common sense dictates that when patients mention their religious faith directly, it is likely that spirituality and their faith community are important to them. While taking a history or in other patient encounters, when significant spiritual or faith issues are noted, clinicians should take a spiritual history. Spirituality should be assessed routinely as part of a social history for outpatient complete physical examinations and for all patients admitted to the hospital.[11,12]

Taking a spiritual history as a routine part of the social history makes it less controversial for some patients, and opens the door to an important aspect of patients' lives that otherwise might not be addressed. Taking a spiritual history is particularly important in hospitalized patients because spiritual issues become more important as patients become more critically ill. Information about spiritual beliefs may give providers insight into patients' medical problems; taking a spiritual history communicates to the patient that the clinician is interested in the patient as a unique individual (see Case 6.2).

Case 6.2

Mrs. J. was a sixty-three-year-old admitted to the hospital from the emergency department because of the inability to walk. Her family had brought her in after she did not report to breakfast that morning. She said she could not move either of her legs; she complained of a mild headache and seemed somewhat depressed. She had a past medical history of hypertension and diet-controlled diabetes. Her social history was stable; she lived with her daughter and son-in-law and got along well with them. Her physical examination showed a normal cardiac and lung exam. Her head, neck, and upper extremities were normal with no neurologic deficit. Her legs had 1+ reflexes bilaterally and no pathologic reflexes. She exhibited some muscle tone when asked to move her legs but was unable to lift her legs off of the bed. A CT scan of the head was normal.

The medical team was strongly considering a diagnosis of conversion reaction. The medical intern returned after morning rounds to interview the patient further. Mrs. J. had lived with her daughter for three years since her husband died. She had another daughter who lived in the same town. She did not smoke, drink alcohol, or use drugs. She denied any conflicts with family members. She had no history of depression or other psychiatric illness.

(continued)

(continued)

The medical intern then asked her whether she had any religious or spiritual beliefs. She immediately became tearful and responded that she was a Methodist. The intern asked whether she belonged to a specific congregation, and she replied that she did, naming the Community Methodist Church. She had been a Christian since she was a child; she and her husband had faithfully participated in church activities for many years. She then admitted that she was upset because she had not continued her financial obligation to the church recently; she believed in "tithing" 10 percent of income to the church. The intern asked whether she would like to speak to a chaplain or her minister, and she responded that she would like to speak with the hospital chaplain. She spoke with the chaplain that afternoon.

The next day the patient was able to bear weight on her legs and walk, and she was discharged from the hospital.

Questions for Discussion:

1. What does this case illustrate about the usefulness of taking a spiritual history? What might have been the consequences if the patient's spiritual concerns had not been addressed?
2. What was the intervention in this case? When can opening a dialogue be therapeutic?

Patients who are admitted to intensive care, facing surgery, or have severe psychiatric illness often have more religious and spiritual concerns. [6-11] For these patients, a spiritual history is paramount. Patients who have terminal conditions also should have a spiritual history taken.[13-16] For example, patients who are facing decisions about active treatment versus hospice care may be weighing concerns about the value of life and the suffering and pain associated with further treatment. Often such decisions are based on the patient's value system and spiritual beliefs as much as on medical prognostic factors (see Chapter 9). Further, whenever resuscitation status of patients is discussed, it is helpful to have prior knowledge about the patient's spiritual beliefs, religious denomination, and faith traditions. For example, many modern Jews do not have definite views of life after death.[17] Clinicians might not be offering comfort to such patients by talking about the patient "leaving this world" for a pleasant life in heaven. On the other hand, belief in an afterlife is a strong component of most Christian denominations and can be a source of comfort for patients who are grieving about a seriously ill or terminally ill loved one. Getting to know patients well and being familiar with their family, social environment, and spiritual context are important aspects of the doctor-patient relationship and a basis for good communications at times of critical medical decision making.

Patient spiritual assessment should be done:
   1. *Whenever religious or spiritual issues are mentioned by the patient*
   2. *Routinely as part of the social history*
   3. *Whenever patients are admitted to the hospital*
   4. *When patients become seriously or terminally ill*

HOW TO TAKE A SPIRITUAL HISTORY

Taking a spiritual history is the process of gathering information from patients about their values, religious beliefs, belief in God, and whatever gives their life meaning. In the clinical context, it also includes questions about how the patients' spiritual views affect their views of illness and health. Often, patients' beliefs are derived from religious foundations, but other times they are based on self, family, nature, or other transcendent values.

Questions should be open-ended at first and become more specific as the history taking progresses. Maugans[12] has developed a tool for taking a spiritual history, SPIRIT, and recommends beginning with the patient's spiritual belief system (Table 6.1). He first asks the patient to describe his or her spiritual belief system. One may also start by asking whether the patient has a religious affiliation. Many patients will describe their beliefs further at this point, others will need to be prompted to provide details of their beliefs.

An assessment of the importance of spirituality in patients' daily life can guide the clinician in probing for more specific beliefs. Reviewing patients' personal involvement in spirituality may illuminate differences in patients' views compared to the views of their formal religious affiliation, i.e., personal views of use of contraception compared to those of the Catholic Church, or views on abortion compared to those of the Church of Christ.

TABLE 6.1. Sample Questions for the SPIRITual History

Mnemonic	Questions
S-Spiritual belief system	What is your formal religious affiliation?
	Name or describe your spiritual belief system.
P-Personal spirituality	Describe the beliefs and practices of your religion or spiritual system that you personally accept.
	Describe the beliefs or practices you do not accept.
	Do you accept or believe . . . (specific tenet or practice)?
	What does your spirituality/religion mean to you?
	What is the importance of your spirituality/religion in daily life?
I-Integration with a spiritual community	Do you belong to any spiritual or religious group or community?
	What is your position or role?
	What importance does this group have to you?
	Is it a source of support? In what ways?
	Does or could this group provide help in dealing with health issues?
R-Ritualized Practices and Restrictions	Are there any specific practices that you carry out as part of your religion/spirituality (e.g., prayer or meditation)?
	Are there certain lifestyle activities or practices that your religion/spirituality encourages or forbids? Do you comply?
	What significance do these practices and restrictions have to you?
	Are there specific elements of medical care that you forbid on the basis or religious/spiritual grounds?
I-Implications	What aspects of your religion/spirituality would you like me to keep in mind as I care for you?
	Would you like to discuss religious or spiritual implications of health care?
	What knowledge or understanding would strengthen our relationship as physician and patient?
	Are there any barriers to our relationship based on religious or spiritual issues?
T-Terminal events planning	As we plan for your care near the end of life, how does your faith impact on your decisions?
	Are there particular aspects of care that you wish to forgo or have withheld because of your faith?

Source: Maugans,T.A. The SPIRITual History. *Archives of Family Medicine,* 1996, 5(1):11-16. Reprinted with permission.

Clinicians should ask about involvement in a church, synagogue, or faith community. Such communities often offer social and spiritual support that is important to patients facing medical illness. Patients may have counseling relationships with clergy in the faith community of which the clinician should be aware. Many religions incorporate behavioral rituals and restrictions into their teaching that affect health. Asking patients about dietary, behavioral, and other restrictions will help clinicians to understand patients better. Sample questions are shown in Table 6.1.

Assessing the implications for medical care of patients' spiritual beliefs is a challenging and ongoing process. As the patients face medical decisions about abortion, contraception, and use of blood transfusions, the implications of patients' religious and spiritual views may become more apparent. Compassion, understanding, and having a spiritual history as a foundation will help clinicians assist patients who are faced with such medical decisions. End-of-life planning is an especially critical time in patients' lives that requires deeper understanding of spiritual issues faced by patients.[13,15]

Several other methods are available to gain the appropriate spiritual information about patients' religious beliefs and spiritual concerns. Perhaps one of the earliest is Kasl's Religious Index[18] (Table 6.2).

Kasl's Religious Index is simple and direct. The questions address three of the most important issues regarding patients' religious and spiritual experience: their attendance at regular religious services (an indicator of religious commitment and predictor of health outcomes); self-assessment of strength of religiousness; and an assessment of religious commitment as a source of strength and comfort.

Although the questions do not address all the issues related to a patient's religiousness and spirituality, they have been used for research in this area for the past decade and a half.

FICA

The FICA assessment (Table 6.3) opens the door to further discussions about spiritual concerns if these are relevant to the patients.[19] Advantages of this tool are its brevity and flexibility for use in different clinical settings.

TABLE 6.2. Kasl's Religious Index

Circle or check the item most descriptive of you in each of the next three questions	
1.	How often do you attend regular religious services during the year? a. Never b. Major holidays only c. More than four times per year d. Weekly e. More than once per week
2.	How religious do you consider yourself to be? a. Religious b. Fairly religious c. Only slightly religious d. Not at all religious e. Against religion
3.	How much is religion (or God) a source of strength and comfort to you? a. Not very much b. Somewhat c. Quite a bit d. A great deal

Source: Adapted from Zuckerman, D.M., Kasl, S.V., Ostfeld, A.M. *American Journal of Epidemiology*, 1984, 119(3):410-423.

Many other indexes have been developed to assess patients' religious and spiritual issues. Most were developed for research and are not practical for regular use by clinicians who have busy office practices and numerous hospitalized patients. Descriptions of two of the most clinically useful instruments are included in this chapter.

The question about faith (F) can be asked in different ways. "What is your faith tradition?" can also be expressed as "What is your religious preference?" Or, in combination with the second question, "Do you have a faith or religion that is important to you?" The question can be customized to different populations of patients by using the terms "faith tradition" or "religious affiliation."

TABLE 6.3. FICA Spiritual Assessment Tool

F-Faith	What is your faith tradition?
I-Important	How important is your faith to you?
C-Church	What is your church or community of faith?
A-Apply/Address	How do your religious and spiritual beliefs apply to your health? How might we address your spiritual needs?

Source: Adapted from Puchalski, C.M. Taking a spiritual history: FICA. *Spirituality and Medicine Connection,* 1999, 3(1):1.

The question about the importance of the patient's faith (I) is critical because it helps the patient express any religious or spiritual concerns. The question from Kasl's Religious Index, "How often do you attend religious services?" can also be asked as a follow-up question. Related questions may be used, such as, "Do you have any religious or spiritual concerns you would like us to address while you are in the hospital?"

The question about church or faith community (C) usually can be asked directly. In the Bible-belt South the question may be asked, "What church do you attend?" Church attendance is so prevalent in that region that even those who do not attend church are used to being asked. In other populations, such as in the Northeast or Pacific Northwest, such a direct question about church may not be appropriate; "Are you a part of a faith community or congregation?" may be preferable. Clinicians may ask a follow-up question regarding specific denomination or a particular church. Knowledge of the beliefs of prominent community congregations may provide insight into the patient's religious and spiritual beliefs. An important follow-up question is whether the church is a source of support for the patient and his or her family.

The question about how beliefs apply to health (A) will uncover restrictions regarding such issues as blood transfusions (Jehovah's Witnesses), rituals such as last rites or communion, and other applications of religious beliefs to health. Clinicians who are more proactive may feel comfortable in asking whether the patient would like the physician or staff members to pray with him or her, or whether the patient would like to be referred to the chaplain or to other pastoral services or counseling. The question about how religious beliefs apply to health may facilitate discussions about end-of-life issues and referrals to hospice care. The "A" in the FICA also may be a reminder to ask the patient, "How would you like us to *address* your faith or spiritual needs while you are in the hospital (or office)"?

MERIT

The MERIT tool is easy to remember (see Table 6.4) and addresses many faith and spiritual issues, including membership in a church or a particular faith tradition (M), and belief in the existence of a higher being (E). It may be just as important to find out about patients who do not believe in a higher being, since they may lack coping resources such as prayer, faith, and a church community. Religious denomination (R) is straightforward. Importance of religion (I) in your life can be rated 1 to 5 or 1 to 10, and is a starting point for asking about spiritual beliefs as they relate to health beliefs, such as contraception or end-of-life planning. The (T) for talk about it further is an important reminder and is similar to the "A" of FICA ("How do your religious beliefs apply to your health?") in that it allows the clinician to ask the patient whether he or she would like to be referred to a chaplain, have prayer, or address spiritual concerns in some other way.

TABLE 6.4. MERIT: A Patient Assessment Tool

M	Member of a church or assembly of worship
E	Existence of a higher being
R	Religious denomination
I	Importance of religion in your life
T	Talk about it further

Source: Donné Thomas-Patterson MD, ECU Brody School of Medicine, 1998. Used by permission.

SUMMARY

Spirituality is an integral part of patients' lives that is often expressed as religiousness. Patients' spirituality should be addressed in the clinical setting because spiritual and religious views affect health, spiritual needs often surface during illness, and spiritual resources may provide assistance in coping with serious illness. Clinicians should take a spiritual history as part of the routine history and physical examination. A more extensive spiritual assessment should be done whenever patients are admitted to the hospital or become terminally ill. Maugans' SPIRITual history, Kasl's Religious Index, Puchalski's FICA tool, and others offer different approaches to assist in obtaining spiritual information from patients. Obtaining such information from patients will be helpful in understanding patients better, addressing patients' spiritual needs, and referring patients for spiritual counseling.

QUESTIONS FOR DISCUSSION

1. When should clinicians seek information about patients' spiritual beliefs and concerns?
2. How can spiritual information from patients be used in clinical care?
3. Describe the FICA spiritual assessment tool and how it could be used in clinical encounters.

Chapter 7

Ethics of Involvement
in Patients' Spirituality

CHAPTER OBJECTIVES

1. To review the salient ethical issues of being involved in patients' spirituality
2. To review the ethical issues involved in collaborating with chaplains
3. To review the ethics of deeper spiritual involvement with patients

INTRODUCTION

Ethics is the branch of philosophy that deals with morality and moral obligations based on rational thought and reason. Medical ethics deals with the duties, responsibilities, and actions of physicians and other caregivers regarding their patients. The role of religion in ethics and medicine is the subject of recent debate.[1-5] The extent to which physicians and other caregivers should become involved in patients' religious or spiritual concerns has not been fully explored. It is important to examine the ethical issues of spiritual involvement, because many health professionals may be reluctant to conduct spiritual assessments and referrals due to ethical considerations. That reluctance has contributed over the past twenty to thirty years to the prevailing attitude that religion and medicine are separate institutions, and that the two should not be intertwined.[6] Some physicians have cautioned against any further in-

tegration of spirituality into clinical medicine due to ethical considerations, while others have promoted more spiritual involvement.[6-9]

One of the central ideas presented in this text is the importance of
understanding and considering patients' spiritual values. Are taking a
spiritual history, being sensitive to spiritual concerns, and referral to
chaplains appropriate responses to considering patients' values? How
should physicians respond to requests to pray with patients? Is it
appropriate to encourage patients to "adopt" spirituality for its health
benefits? Addressing the ethics of spiritual involvement is essential to
providing morally and spiritually appropriate clinical care.

ETHICS OF SPIRITUAL INQUIRY

The first step in addressing the ethics of spiritual involvement is
determining whether it is ethically acceptable to inquire about patients'
religious and spiritual beliefs. This determination should be based on
the importance of obtaining the information and the rights and responsibilities of physicians and patients. Any inquiry should respect patients' basic rights of autonomy, confidentiality, and privacy.

Obtain Important Information

Obtaining important medical information is one ethical justification for spiritual inquiry. Jamison has pointed out that most disease
and injury result from lifestyle choices rooted in cultural personal
values rather than distinct organic pathology.[7] He goes further to
express that ignoring the spiritual dimension of human beings is on
a par with making a diagnosis without an adequate physical examination. Wind[8] has supported the inclusion of religion in dealing
with bioethics and medical decision making because it produces a
more accurate view of the people encountered in the health care
setting. Spiritual inquiry may be justified on the basis of obtaining
important and accurate information regarding patients' health, health
beliefs, and personal behaviors that affect health.

A counterargument is that inquiring about patients' spiritual concerns is inherently "nonmedical" and therefore outside the realm of
acceptable disclosure. Sloan and colleagues[9] have raised this con-

cern, saying that physicians should not promote a nonmedical agenda, and that to do so would abuse their status as professionals. They object specifically to making inquiries into a patient's spiritual life for the purpose of making recommendations that link religious practice with better outcomes. Sloan does make an allowance for "taking into account" religious factors, so that basic inquiry would be ethical, but not inquiry leading to nonmedical or spiritual interventions.

Rights and Responsibilities

The concept of rights and responsibilities of physicians and patients can be applied to spiritual inquiry. Physicians claim the right to inquire about spiritual concerns that may have an impact on health or health beliefs. Patients have the right to respond to such inquiry, respond within certain limits, or decline. A survey of physicians and patients in Vermont[10] investigated the rights and responsibilities of religious inquiry. In that study, 89 percent of physicians and 52 percent of patients agreed with the *right* of the physician to inquire about religion and religious concerns; 52 percent of physicians and 21 percent of patients felt it was the *responsibility* of the physician to inquire. This study may reflect attitudes of people in only one region, but it does illustrate the divided views of physicians and patients regarding religious inquiry. Whether use of the term "spiritual" rather than "religious" inquiry would have made a difference in the results of the survey is unknown.

Patient Autonomy, Privacy, and Confidentiality

Patient autonomy in the physician/patient encounter implies that patients have the right to make choices independently of physicians. Physicians are providers of information and may recommend particular tests, treatments, or referrals. Although complete objectivity is the ideal, clinicians are aware that their biases and backgrounds affect their recommendations. Some patients may consider any inquiry into spiritual matters an inherently biased interaction that imposes on their autonomy.

Spiritual inquiry also may be considered an invasion of privacy. People who follow different faith traditions have different views regarding the degree that religious concerns should be discussed in public. Physicians may respond that private religious views in such areas as abortion and euthanasia affect medical decisions and are therefore relevant to the medical encounter. Patients may prefer that physicians address their viewpoint without inquiring about the religious or spiritual basis for it. When the patient's desire for privacy conflicts with the clinician's need to obtain important medical information, compassionate understanding of the relevance of spiritual issues will help in negotiating a solution.

Patients' desire for confidentiality extends to religious and spiritual information that is shared in the medical interview. Just as health professionals hold in confidence any medical history obtained, so should they hold in confidence any spiritual history, unless given permission by the patient to share such information outside the medical team.

Obtaining information about patients' religious and spiritual beliefs may be ethically justified because of the importance of obaining pertinent medical information. Physicians believe they have the right to take a spiritual assessment. Patients ethically demand that spiritual inquiry respect their autonomy, privacy, and confidentiality.

ETHICS OF REFERRAL TO CHAPLAINS

Davis[11] has said that health care providers should be knowledgeable about the religious and cultural values of people they treat. Culturally and spiritually sensitive providers may discover significant spiritual or religious concerns in patients that relate to health. Once such issues are identified, the provider must decide how best to address them, including dealing with them personally, ignoring them, asking the patient to address them, or seeking consultation. Many providers feel uncomfortable inquiring about religious and spiritual concerns; even fewer would feel qualified and prepared to counsel patients directly about such matters. Although many such issues may have been ignored in the past, the well-trained clinician should be able to assess patients' concerns and then refer the patient to a certified chaplain (see Chapter 8, "Chaplains and Pastoral Services") or other qualified spiritual counselor.

Thiel and Robinson[12] have proposed that physicians routinely collaborate with chaplains and regularly refer patients to them. They present a broadened biopsychosocial model that regularly includes the realm of the spiritual. Their reasoning is that patients would be better served by physicians who regularly incorporate spiritual and religious concerns into patient assessment, and recommend consulting with chaplains when spiritual needs outside the competence of the physician are identified. Chaplains offer expertise and experience in spiritual counseling that physicians do not possess; using more qualified professionals should improve the quality of care. Most referrals to chaplains come from nurses or social workers, rather than physicians. If one agrees that it is an obligation of physicians to inquire about spiritual concerns that relate to health, and such concerns are identified, then it seems the ethics and professionalism of the physician should compel him or her to seek assistance from a chaplain. Further, most patients facing serious medical illness feel religion is important in their medical care.[6,10] Some patients prefer to address their spiritual concerns with a physician, others prefer a chaplain or other minister.[10,13]

Experimental evidence supports chaplain use and referral. One study of open-heart surgery patients found that those randomly referred to a supplementary chaplain intervention recovered more quickly and required two fewer hospital days than control patients.[14] Another study found that orthopedic surgery patients needed less pain medication when receiving daily chaplain visits.[15] If collaboration between physicians and chaplains broadens the biopsychosocial model, is welcomed by patients, and is empirically beneficial to health, then the ethics of such collaboration have much to commend it.

The counterargument is that religious ground is hallowed ground, and should not be broached by physicians. Referral to chaplains may make the patient uncomfortable; the authoritative position of the physician may deter the patient from objecting. A subtle coercion to "go along" with religious or spiritual actions or commitments may take place that would compromise the patient's integrity and perhaps build mistrust between the physician and the patient. Adding a burden of guilt to patients who may feel "unworthy" spiritually, and who are already physically ill, may actually harm, not help patients.[9]

Chaplain referral is ethically appropriate when clinicians identify patients with spiritual beliefs or concerns that go beyond their expertise. Sensitivity to the patient's autonomy and integrity is paramount.

ETHICS OF PRAYER WITH PATIENTS

How should physicians respond to a request to pray with patients? Whether it is ethical to participate in prayer with patients is a question that physicians may have to face. Forty-eight percent of inpatients in one study said they want their physician to pray with them.[13] The 1990 Gallup poll (Religion in America) found that 76 percent of respondents mostly or completely agreed that prayer is an important part of daily life. Another study found that 96 percent of patients awaiting heart surgery used prayer to cope with their stress.[16] A patient-initiated request to pray seems to eliminate many of the ethical objectives to physician involvement; since the physician is responding to an invitation, the involvement cannot be construed as coercive or not respecting the patient's privacy or autonomy. Physician discomfort with the situation can be overcome with training and experience.

Although some physicians may pray privately for patients, or listen while the patient prays, fewer would initiate prayer. Many physicians are concerned about imposing their own beliefs on patients or feel they have not been properly trained to initiate spiritual involvement.[17] Maugans[18] has described prayer with patients as common and appropriate, whether initiated by the patient or in response to a noncoercive offer by a physician. Such activity may enhance the doctor-patient relationship, especially when both parties have the same or similar religious beliefs.[19]

The counterargument is that patients may feel forced to comply with any physician request and may be uncomfortable objecting for fear of biasing further treatment by the physician. The subtle coercion of an invitation to pray is not easily refused by patients. Patients may also feel their autonomy or privacy is threatened because of pressure to reveal privately held religious or spiritual beliefs. They may believe that religion and medicine are separate, and that the separation should remain intact. Others may prefer to address spiritual issues with their minister, rabbi, or other religious leaders, rather than physicians. Patients always retain the right to decline to participate in prayer or decline referral to a chaplain.

Patient-initiated prayer respects patients' autonomy and should invite physician response. Physicians may consider offering to pray with patients if it is done in a noncoercive way that respects religious and spiritual beliefs.

SUMMARY

This chapter offers guidance to clinicians who are considering the ethics of spiritual involvement in clinical practice. Clinicians should address whether it is ethically appropriate to take a spiritual history, refer to chaplains, and pray with patients. Taking a history may be justified by the need to obtain important information that may affect health, but needs to be done in a way that respects patients' rights of autonomy, privacy, and confidentiality. Patients should be referred to chaplains or other ministers when significant spiritual concerns or needs are identified. Patients who initiate prayer are inviting a response from physicians and other health professionals. Physicians who initiate prayer with patients who have similar religious beliefs may enhance the doctor-patient relationship. Patients have the right to refuse participation in spiritual counseling, prayer, or spiritual inquiry.

QUESTIONS FOR DISCUSSION

1. Do physicians have a right to inquire about patients' spiritual concerns? Religious beliefs?

2. Do physicians have an obligation to inquire about spiritual or religious beliefs? How does the epidemiological association between religious commitment and better health affect this obligation?
3. Should physicians refer patients to chaplains routinely? Should all patients in the intensive care unit and the cancer ward be required to talk with a chaplain?
4. What problems have you seen when patients are referred to chaplains?
5. What is the relationship of physicians and chaplains at your hospital? Does your hospital have a chaplain residency program? Do chaplains participate in rounds with the medical or surgical teams?
6. How should health professionals respond to a request to pray with a patient?
7. Should health professionals offer to pray with patients? For patients?
8. Should physicians cite the epidemiologic evidence for improved health outcomes with greater religious involvement when counseling patients about personal health risks? Should physicians divulge their own religious affiliation to patients? If so, in what situations?

CASES FOR DISCUSSION

Case 7.1

You are a physician caring for a seventy-six-year-old woman, Mrs. K, who is terminally ill and on a ventilator. In your best clinical judgment, you can do nothing more for Mrs. K, and you feel that life support is only prolonging her suffering. You suggest to the family that she be allowed to die naturally and peacefully. Mrs. K's daughter responds that she believes God will cure her, and that she should remain on the ventilator until God sees fit to do so. Further, she says she has seen God act in the lives of others. What would you say to Mrs. K's daughter? How would you respond to a request to pray with her? What would you say if she asked you to accompany her to a faith-healing service at her church?

Case 7.2

You are a physician in private practice. You are also a committed Christian and an elder in the First Baptist Church in your town. You are caring for Mr. Y, a middle-aged man recovering from injuries suffered in a motor vehicle accident while driving under the influence of alcohol. Mr. Y has many social and emotional problems, including mild depression and a strained marital relationship. He also tells you he was raised as a Baptist, but has not attended church in many years. You have recently read an article about sharing your faith,[19] and feel that Mr. Y would greatly benefit from a return to regular church attendance. Would it be appropriate for you to suggest that he start attending church again? Why or why not? Should you suggest instead that he seek counseling from a pastor? How would you respond if he asked why you were recommending this?

Case 7.3

You are a family physician in private practice. Mr. J, a thirty-five-year-old college professor, comes to you with swelling and pain in the knee. You diagnose an effusion, and recommend X rays and anti-inflammatory medication. Mr. J makes it clear that he does not want "artificial" medicine, since he believes we are polluting our bodies and the planet with toxins. He would prefer a "natural" or "alternative" remedy that is environmentally friendly. When you try to explain, you discover that he holds a quite coherent, but in your opinion, misguided set of beliefs about being in harmony with the natural world. Although you accept that Mr. J's belief system is spiritual, albeit not religious, and that it guides his choices and actions in much the same way as a religion, in your considered judgment he is harming himself by refusing your prescription. What would you do? You suggest a consultation with the chaplain but the patient refuses. What else could you do? What if he had been in a more serious accident and suffered an injury that required an operation and blood transfusion, but he declined because blood from others is "unnatural"?

Chapter 8

Chaplains and Pastoral Services

CHAPTER OBJECTIVES

1. To review the education and training of chaplains
2. To review the role of the chaplain in the interdisciplinary care of patients
3. To review the impact of pastoral care on health

INTRODUCTION

Chaplains are ministers trained to work in medical and clinical settings. They provide religious, spiritual, and emotional support to patients and their families. Support may include pastoral counseling, ministry to persons of diverse cultural and religious backgrounds, assessment of patients' spiritual needs, grief counseling, patient and family visitation, end-of-life care, participation in interdisciplinary patient care rounds, and other duties. Chaplains are usually employed by the hospital, although some are volunteers. Usual hours of availability are 8 a.m. to 5 p.m., Monday through Friday. Most chaplains provide evening and weekend services on a rotating or "on call" basis. An example of typical pastoral services offered at larger hospitals is shown in Figure 8.1. Chaplains often serve on hospital and departmental ethics committees and boards. Many are members of the Association of Professional Chaplains (APC), a not-for-profit professional association (see Figure 8.2).

EDUCATION AND TRAINING

Chaplains must hold an undergraduate degree from an accredited college or university. The undergraduate degree can be in any major, although most chaplains hold degrees in the arts and sciences.

FIGURE 8.1. Clinical Pastoral Services

UC**DAVIS**
HEALTH SYSTEM

Clinical Pastoral Services
UC Davis Medical Center
(916) 734-3657

Housestaff Building, Room 1002
2315 Stockton Boulevard
Sacramento, California 95817

The purpose of Clinical Pastoral Services is to provide in-depth spiritual comfort, guidance, support, counseling for patients, their families and staff in times of physical, emotional, and spiritual crisis.

As members of the health care team chaplains are available:

To offer comfort;
To listen and explore personal resources;
To provide counseling, prayer, and/or sacraments;
To provide pastoral support;
To discuss Advance Directives;
To help clarify ethical decisions and concerns;
Or, if you just need someone with whom to talk, a chaplain will listen!

Please call 734-3657, Monday through Friday, 8 a.m. to 5 p.m. to request a visit. Service on evenings and weekends is provided on call and can be requested through the nursing staff or by contacting the hospital operator at 734-2011. A Catholic chaplain is available and can be reached on pager 762-5507.

UC Davis Health System sponsors a Clinical Pastoral Education program. The CPE program is accredited by the Association for Clinical Pastoral Education and trains students in hospital chaplaincy. For more information about the program, please call 734-3657.

UC Davis Medical Center Community Relations Homepage

Community Relations oversees several other departments, Medical Interpreting Services, Patient Relations, and Volunteer Services (which itself is responsible for Clinical Pastoral Services, Lifeline, the Child's Play Center, and the Gift Shop and is liaison to the Kiwanis Family House).

Thank you for your interest in Clinical Pastoral services at UC Davis Medical Center!

Source:http://web.ucdme.ucdavis.edu/PastoralServices/, UC Davis Web site, October 13, 1999. Reprinted with permission.

FIGURE 8.2. Core Values of the Association of Professional Chaplains

1. The individual person possesses dignity and worth.
2. The spiritual dimension is an essential part of an individual's striving for health and meaning in life.
3. The spiritual care of persons is a critical aspect of the total care offered in the delivery of care for public and private institutions and organizations.
4. Inclusivity and diversity are seen as foundational values in pastoral services offered to persons, regardless of religion, race, ethnicity, sexual orientation, age, disability, or gender. Inclusivity and diversity are also valued throughout the structure of the Association.
5. Public advocacy, related to spiritual values and social justice concerns, is promoted on behalf of persons in need.

Source: The Association of Professional Chaplains, 1998.

Board certification requires additional theological education at the graduate professional level, usually at least three years at an accredited institution. A summary of the Master of Arts in clinical ministry program at Loma Linda University is shown in Figure 8.3. Program requirements for the Master of Arts (MA) in clinical ministry are shown in Figure 8.4.

Hospital chaplains undergo an additional year of training in a clinical pastoral care residency at an acute care hospital. Certification as a hospital chaplain also requires being ordained or commissioned by a religious organization. Ordination is recognition of commitment to ministry after recommendation from peers. An additional requirement for certification is ecclesiastical endorsement by a faith group for ministry in a specialized setting. Board certification is granted by the APC after receipt of required letters of recommendation and documentation of completion of clinical pastoral education. The APC offers associate chaplain status to ordained ministers with two years of graduate training.

Clinical pastoral education expands knowledge in theology and the behavioral sciences. Training also promotes the ability to establish meaningful relationships with peers and hospital personnel, to work creatively, and to facilitate the spiritual growth of persons of

FIGURE 8.3. Master of Arts in Clinical Ministry

The master of arts in clinical ministry prepares students for integrating spirituality and healing within the health care professions, as well as other ministries. It is designed for three types of students: those seeking to pursue graduate studies in religion and/or ministry; those wishing to enhance already existing careers with graduate study in religion and ministry; and those willing to use this degree as a stepping stone to doctoral study.

This degree furthers the educational process of caring for the whole person through the development of clinical skills. It blends two major areas of concentration: academic preparation and clinical experience.

The faculty represent a balance between academic expertise and clinical experience, as well as a variety of disciplines including biblical studies, theology, practical theology, marriage and family therapy, cultural psychology, American church history, health education, nursing, and ethics.

As a premier teaching and research hospital, Loma Linda University Medical Center is in an excellent setting for the clinical aspects of this program.

Source: http://www.llu/edu/llu/ministry/index.html, Loma Linda University Web site, July 22, 1999. Reprinted with permission.

diverse backgrounds. It is important for hospital chaplains to be trained in crisis counseling and grief counseling. They also must be able to demonstrate thorough knowledge of theological concepts and relate to patients with compassion and understanding without denominational bias.

Chaplains are specially trained ministers with graduate-level education in theology, counseling, and behavioral science. Many achieve certification by the Association of Professional Chaplains.

ROLE OF THE CHAPLAIN

In addition to providing grief counseling, assessment of patients' spiritual needs, and dealing with patients' end-of-life issues, chaplains also provide support to hospital staff (see Photo 8.5). Medical and nursing staff may need pastoral support during or following critical

FIGURE 8.4. Program Requirements for the MA in Clinical Ministry at Loma Linda University

LOMA LINDA UNIVERSITY

Faculty of Religion
MA in Clinical Ministry
Program requirements

In order to receive the master of arts in clinical ministry from Loma Linda University, each student will:

1. Complete a minimum of 48 units of course work as herein specified with an overall grade point average of B or better, with no grade lower than C, and with no grade in a core course lower than a B-. The required curriculum is as follows:

Core: (36-48 units)

RELR 565	Introduction to Ministry in Institutional Settings	3-4
RELR 567	Introduction to Pastoral Counseling	3-4
RELR 568	Care of the Dying and Bereaved	3-4
RELR 574	Preaching Practicum in Clinical Ministry	3-4
RELR 584	Culture, Psychology, & Religion	3-4
RELR 694	Seminar in Clinical Ministry	3-4
RELF 557	A Theology of Human Suffering	3-4
RELF 558	Old Testament Theology	3-4
RELF 559	New Testament Theology	3-4
RELE 504	Research Methods	3-4
RELE 524	Christian Bioethics	3-4
MF AM 515	Crisis Intervention Counseling	3

General: (0-12 units)

Selectives in order to complete a minimum of 48 units, offered by the Faculty of Religion and/or other departments and schools within LLU.

TOTAL	48 units

2. Be permitted to transfer up to eight units of approved graduate-level courses from other institutions into LLU's program in clinical ministry.

3. Satisfactorily complete an approved one year (i.e., 1,600 hours) clinical internship. The program recommends that this requirement be met by the satisfactory completion of four quarters of Clinical Pastoral Education at an

FIGURE 8.4 *(continued)*

accredited C.P.E. center. (Note: Acceptance into a quarter of C.P.E. is at the discretion of the C.P.E. supervisor and must be arranged individually and in advance.)

The expectation of the program is that all students will complete all course work before entering the clinical internship. In rare cases, however, a student may petition the director of the program to take the clinical internship out of sequence. Even in such cases, the recommendation is that certain classes, namely RELR 565, RELR 568, and RELR 694, be completed before entering the clinical internship.

C.P.E. (RELR 524), if taken as a selective, may account for a maximum of six academic units, and, if taken for academic credit, must be taken in addition to the 1,600-hour clinical internship.

After every 400-hour segment, a clinical evaluation form must be submitted to the program director.

4. Pass comprehensive written examinations. These examinations will test the student's ability to integrate and apply knowledge from the overall program. These examinations must be successfully completed before the student defends a thesis or its approved substitute.

5. Either prepare a thesis while registered for RELR 698 or prepare two major papers of publishable quality in courses approved as substitutes by the guidance committee. The student must provide an oral defense of a thesis or two major papers that analyze specific issues, cases, or themes in clinical ministry. Students must declare whether they intend to write a thesis by the time they complete 12 quarter units in the program.

6. Individual variations from these requirements may be permitted by special request for faculty review.

Source: http://www.llu/edu/ministry/llufrcmr2.htm, Loma Linda University Web site, October 13, 1999. Reprinted with permission.

incidents such as an unexpected or life-threatening event. Chaplains also serve as consultants to staff regarding patients' religious beliefs and provide staff and patient advocacy.

The patient, the nursing staff, the medical staff, or others may request support from hospital chaplains. In certain specialized clinical areas, contact with the chaplain may be routine, such as in neonatal intensive care units or cancer wards. In other areas, chaplains provide services when requested.

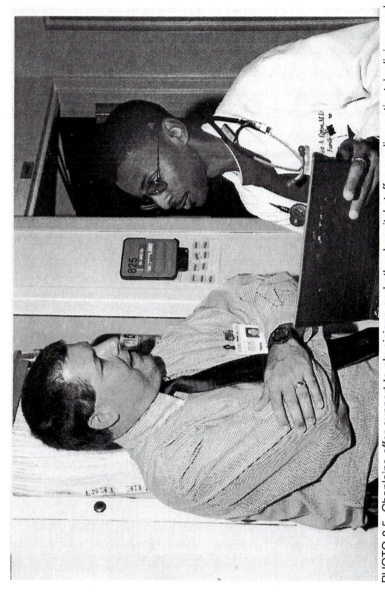

PHOTO 8.5. Chaplains offer support to physicians and other hospital staff regarding patients' religious and spiritual beliefs. Photograph by Margaret Atwood, MUSC Art Services and Digital Imaging. Reprinted with permission of MUSC.

Chaplains also provide direct services to patients, families, and staff.[1] They offer prayer with and for patients; conduct worship services, memorial services, and sacramental services; provide religious literature; and coordinate communications with patients' home religious communities. Chaplains also provide educational services for staff and clergy in a variety of settings. They often provide community outreach education for clergy regarding pastoral care in the hospital setting. Chaplains often serve as leaders or coordinators of support groups for patients with various illnesses.

End-of-life care and ethical decision making are areas in which chaplains are called upon for consultation and service.[2-3] Chaplains may serve on medical ethics boards as well as on institutional research review boards.

Chaplains provide spiritual and emotional support to patients, families, and hospital staff. They also serve the hospital and community through outreach, education, and leadership of various groups.

COLLABORATING WITH CHAPLAINS IN THE TREATMENT OF PATIENTS

Physicians and other clinical staff are welcome to call upon chaplain services for assistance. Chaplains are prepared to work with medical and nursing staff and others in in dealing with the spiritual and emotional issues of health, assessing patients' spiritual needs, and counseling.[2-4]

For example, physicians have often informed patients of the diagnosis of cancer without preparing them or their families and without involving others to help patients process their feelings about the diagnosis and its implications. Most chaplains would welcome the opportunity to be present when the diagnosis of cancer is communicated to a patient and collaborate with nurses and physicians in offering spiritual care.[4] Dealing with the diagnosis from the patients' point of view involves far more than the simple facts of the diagnosis, prognosis, and the medical options available for treatment. The emotional devastation of this diagnosis is often underestimated by treating physicians. The word "cancer" means suffering and death to many people. Patients may not hear anything after the word is mentioned and important information communicated by the physician may be lost.

Chaplains can provide a unique supportive role because of their ability to provide not only emotional support but religious and spiritual support as well. Patients often react to the news of the diagnosis of cancer with anger or denial. An experienced chaplain can assist the patient in working through those stages to the level of acceptance (see Case 8.1).[1,3]

Case 8.1

Miss P. was a twenty-five-year-old woman diagnosed with lymphoma and admitted to the hospital for chemotherapy. The physician, who was cross-covering for one of his partners, performed the history and physical examination. The patient previously had experienced one inpatient admission for chemotherapy. She was unmarried, with no children. The physician noted that the patient was apprehensive. She was thin, but not cachectic, with prominent nodes in the neck and axillary areas. Her heart and lung exams were normal.

The physician noted that the patient's family lived in another state, and that Miss P. was from a town two hours away from the hospital. The physician took a spiritual history and learned that Miss P. relied heavily upon her church for emotional and spiritual support. She was anxious about not being able to see her minister while she was in the hospital, due to the long distance from home. The physician referred her to the chaplain.

The chaplain met with Miss P. and listened to her fears about having severe nausea with treatment, her concerns about her worth in God's eyes, and her search for meaning in life now that she had cancer. They shared Scripture about God's sovereignty and love, and prayed together.

Miss P. tolerated the chemotherapy well. Her demeanor was cheery and upbeat, and she visited other patients on the ward to offer words of encouragement. Other physicians on the staff noted her positive disposition; she openly credited her relationship with God, and often joked and laughed with the chaplain during his daily visits.

Questions for Discussion

1. What role did the physician play in addressing the patient's spiritual concerns? What role did the chaplain play?
2. What type of religious coping strategies did the patient use? What are some examples of positive and negative religious coping strategies?
3. What other roles do hospital chaplains play in addition to direct patient counseling?

In addition, physicians may have to present the patient with the diagnosis of cancer, and then proceed to treating other patients in the emergency room or hospital. The chaplain may be able to spend a more extended period of time with the patient initially and make arrangements for follow-up on subsequent days to offer religious, spiritual, and emotional support. Such support often includes prayer and may include other religious ceremonies, such as last rites.

Many diagnoses can have an emotionally devastating effect on the patient, such as the diagnosis of seizure disorder or acquired immuno-deficiency syndrome.[5,6] Diagnoses of less severe illnesses still can lead patients to ask spiritual questions (Why me? What did I do? Is this punishment from God?). Counseling patients regarding medical options or using a psychological approach may not completely address the needs of patients who are considering spiritual questions, such as the meaning of their lives, whether there is life after death, or the meaning of suffering in their lives.[7] Such questions may best be addressed by chaplains, with special knowledge, skills, and training in spiritual issues. Coordinating care/treatment recommendations between chaplains and the medical team is critical to quality care (see Photo 8.6). Conflicting advice from medical and spiritual caregivers can be detrimental to the patient's coping and emotional health. Clinicians who are aware of the specialized education of chaplains are more likely to collaborate with chaplains for the benefit of patients.

Patients often have spiritual needs and concerns that are best addressed by a professional chaplain. Spiritual care should be part of a collaborative team approach in the overall medical care of patients.

THE IMPACT OF PASTORAL CARE ON HEALTH

Whether devoting more attention to people's spiritual needs leads to better health is currently under study. The primary motivation for spiritual care and counseling is to meet spiritual needs, regardless of whether such care also improves physical health. Nevertheless, some researchers have noted improvements in physical health when spiritual needs are addressed. McSherry and colleagues have described a case series in which chaplain visits were part of the total health care

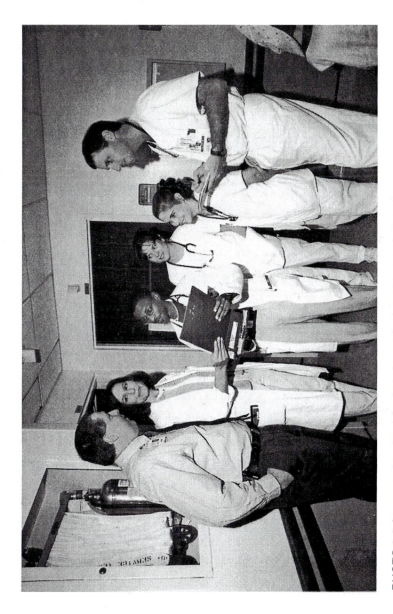

PHOTO 8.6. Incorporating chaplains into the medical team in a multidisciplinary approach enhances coordination and quality of clinical care. Photograph by Margaret Atwood, MUSC Art Services and Digital Imaging. Reprinted with permission of MUSC.

of hospitalized patients.[8] Hospital stays were shortened among patients receiving a chaplain visit. Koenig has reported the findings of a random trial in 700 hospitalized veterans, comparing daily chaplain visits to daily volunteer "cheer-up" visits or usual care.[9] Patients who had received daily chaplain visits exhibited less depression and averaged two fewer days in the hospital compared to the other groups.

The impact of chaplains on care of patients in intensive care also has been studied. Field and colleagues[10] reported on the use of a comprehensive supportive care team that included a physician, a nurse, a social worker, and a chaplain. Their case series described a reduction in intensive care length of stay from twelve days to six days for twenty patients using the intervention team, compared with a similar group treated before the development of the team.

These findings support that pastoral care has an impact beyond meeting patients' spiritual needs. Further research should be done to investigate how a multidisciplinary team approach that includes chaplain care affects medical outcomes in various settings.

SUMMARY

Chaplains undergo graduate education and specialized pastoral care residencies to become certified by the Association of Professional Chaplains. Pastoral education includes theological, behavioral, and counseling curricula. Chaplains offer spiritual and emotional support to seriously ill patients, and can be an important resource for the health care team. A few studies have investigated the impact of chaplain care on health, but further research needs to be done.

QUESTIONS FOR DISCUSSION

1. How many chaplains work at your hospital? What training have they had?
2. How have you seen chaplains participate on the health care team? What is their role in the intensive care unit? The cancer ward?
3. Have you ever made rounds with a chaplain? Were the issues discussed different from those encountered on medical rounds?

Chapter 9

Spirituality in Special Patient Populations: Dying Patients

CHAPTER OBJECTIVES

1. To review the role of spirituality in end-of-life decisions
2. To review the use of spirituality as a coping mechanism for dying patients
3. To review the importance of inquiring about belief in miracles and belief in an afterlife in dying patients

INTRODUCTION

Patients approaching the end of life often have many anxieties and concerns, including concerns about their loved ones and how they will be cared for after they are gone.[1] Such patients also may have terminal cancer, congestive heart failure, arthritis, or other diseases that cause considerable pain and discomfort. Physicians and other health care specialists caring for patients nearing the end of life have been trained to treat pain and assist with medical decision making; some also refer patients for counseling, arrange for living wills, and deal with family issues. Most physicians have not been trained to deal with the profound spiritual issues and concerns that accompany the end of life. Such issues include forgiveness, unresolved conflicts with loved ones, and the patient's beliefs in the afterlife. Failure to deal with spiritual concerns when patients are nearing the end of life can have detrimental consequences, including depression, poor medical decision making, grief, and family conflict.

THE ROLE OF SPIRITUALITY
IN END-OF-LIFE DECISIONS

The role of spirituality in patients' end-of-life decisions has not been fully explored. Spiritual needs of dying patients are not routinely addressed by physicians or the health care team, even though patients' spiritual beliefs often provide the context for end-of-life decisions. Spiritual concerns are among the top concerns of people who express anxiety about dying[1] (see Table 9.1).

In a study of predominantly African-American, Christian, HIV-positive patients, ninety patients were asked about resuscitation status, possession of a living will, and several spiritual factors.[2] Ninety-eight percent believed in God, and 81 percent believed in God's forgiveness. Twenty-six percent of respondents believed their HIV disease was a form of punishment; 17 percent believed it was a punishment from God, and 44 percent felt guilty about their HIV infection. These results illustrate the prevalence of spiritual concerns in one group of terminal patients, and are consistent with the concerns reported in a national survey[1] in which the top spiritual concern was "not being forgiven by God" (Table 9.1). Fear of death was also explored in the study of HIV-positive patients: it was more likely to be found in those who felt guilty about their HIV infection (OR = 2.6, P = 0.014) or who believed HIV was punishment (OR = 3.7, P = 0.010). Fear of death was less likely in those who stated God was part of their purpose in life (OR = .11, P = 0.014), and less likely in those who read the Bible daily, weekly, or monthly (OR = .31, P = .015). Discussions of resuscitation status were more likely among those who believed in God's forgiveness (OR = 6.7, P = 0.043); respondents who prayed daily were 7.9 times more likely (P = 0.025) to possess a living will.

TABLE 9.1 Anxiety About Dying Concerns in Rank Order

Concern (in order of most to least importance)	Percent	Type
The possibility of being vegetable-like for some period of time	73	Medical
Not having the chance to say good-bye to someone	70	Emotional
The possibility of great physical pain before death	67	Medical
How loved ones will be cared for	65	Practical

Concern (in order of most to least importance)	Percent	Type
Thinking that death will be the cause of inconvenience and stress for loved ones	64	Emotional
Not being forgiven by God	56	Spiritual
Not reconciling with others	56	Spiritual
The possibility of not having access to life-saving medical technology	56	Medical
The possibility of not having access to one's own doctor or hospital	52	Medical
Dying when removed or cut off from God or a higher power	51	Spiritual
The possibility of continued emotional suffering	51	Emotional
Not being forgiven by someone for a wrongdoing	49	Spiritual
Having other people make medical decisions	48	Medical
The possibility of being alone when dying	47	Emotional
Not having made or updated a will	43	Practical
Not having completed life work	43	Practical
The idea of being in a hospital if dying	41	Medical
Not having a blessing from a family member or clergyperson	39	Spiritual
What the afterlife will be like	39	Spiritual
Wondering about being missed or remembered over time	35	Emotional
Not being alive and part of this world	32	Emotional
Not having made burial arrangements	32	Practical
Having someone go through possessions after death	19	Practical
What will be said at the funeral	13	Practical

Source: Adapted from George H. Gallup International Institute. Spiritual Beliefs and the Dying Process: A Report on a National Survey. The Nathan Cummings Foundation and Fetzer Institute, October 1997.

These findings have important implications for caring for people who are terminally ill. Spiritual concerns are prevalent among the dying, especially issues of forgiveness and guilt. Spiritual concerns are a significant hindrance to end-of-life planning and should be addressed by the health care team.

Kaldjian and colleagues summarized the implications of their study[2]:

Our results suggest that spiritual beliefs may either enhance or diminish an HIV-positive patient's ability to discuss end-of-life decisions. Physicians should therefore acquaint themselves with those spiritual beliefs of their patients that relate to death in order to identify those beliefs that may facilitate, and those that may impede, the establishment of advance directives . . .

Discussions about resuscitation status are essential to good patient care, but they can be the cause of considerable anxiety and fear. If they are detached from a patient's beliefs and commitments, such discussions may be even more disturbing. If a patient holds spiritual or religious beliefs that provide comfort in the face of death, the physician can assist the patient by using those supportive beliefs to frame a discussion about resuscitative status. If a patient does not hold such beliefs, or if a patient's beliefs cause discomfort, further discussions or referral for spiritual counseling might be appropriate.

The study of HIV-positive patients took place in one defined population in a single community. Whether the beliefs expressed apply to other terminally ill patients is not known. The fact that 90 percent of the patients were Christian limits the generalizability of the findings to other religious and nonreligious groups. Nevertheless, the study's findings may be important to consider when dealing with the large Christian population in the United States. Physicians dealing with patients who are reluctant to address end-of-life issues should consider whether spiritual beliefs or concerns are playing a role.

Physicians should identify the spiritual beliefs of dying patients in order to assess whether those beliefs may impede discussion of end-of-life issues, and refer patients for spiritual counseling when appropriate.

SPIRITUALITY AS A COPING MECHANISM

Fear of death is common in patients with terminal illness.[3] Some patients approach death with great anxiety, others with remorse, and still others with great calm. Spirituality and religious commitment are among the available means of dealing with the tremendous burden of impending death.

A survey of 108 women with gynecologic cancer found that fear was the predominant psychosocial consequence of having cancer.[3] Specified fears were fear of pain (63 percent), dying (56 percent), losing control over their lives (48 percent), and becoming totally dependent (46 percent). Over 75 percent indicated that religion had an important place in their lives; 93 percent felt that religious commitment helped sustain their hopes.

Other researchers have found similar reliance on religious and spiritual coping strategies. Mickley and colleagues[4] found that women with breast cancer who had increased spiritual well-being also felt more hopeful. Gibbs and associates[5] found less fear of death among patients with terminal cancer who had self-professed strong religious beliefs. Ringdal[6] investigated 253 patients with cancer and found that greater religious involvement was associated with greater satisfaction with life and with greater hopefulness. These associations were present after controlling for the potential confounders of age, sex, education level, and stage of illness. Further, in a study by Yates and colleagues,[7] religious commitment and activity were associated with lower levels of pain reported by patients with advanced cancer. A study of 114 adults with cancer[8] found a significant correlation between spiritual well-being and reduced anxiety. It is important to note that the scale used (Ellison Spiritual Well-Being Scale)[9] reflects spiritual peace and "settledness," not strength of beliefs or attendance at religious services. The implication of the data is that spiritual well-being, expressed as feeling a sense of meaning and purpose and feeling connected to a higher being, is an important coping resource in patients with cancer.

Research in this field has not progressed to the point of showing differences in medical outcome after addressing patients' spiritual concerns. However, the importance of religious coping in dying patients is clear. Physicians who assist patients in dealing with terminal illness should be sensitive to the spiritual beliefs and concerns of the patient. Patients may not have the awareness, ability, or strength to resolve such concerns, and may benefit from the physician inquiring about spiritual beliefs. Nearly half of the patients in the HIV study wanted to discuss their spiritual needs with the physician.[2] Whether spiritual counseling or another intervention can help patients achieve a greater sense of spiritual well-being and thus lower anxiety has not been investigated. However, it would appear that acknowledgement of patients' anxiety and heeding patients' requests for referral for spiritual counseling would be appropriate.

Use of religious and spiritual resources represents an important coping strategy in dying patients. Clinicians who are sensitive to spiritual concerns in dying patients will be better able to assist patients nearing the end of life.

BELIEF IN MIRACLES AND AN AFTERLIFE

Belief in miracles is part of the faith tradition of many of the most prevalent religions in the United States, including Christianity, Mormonism, and Judaism. A survey of 1,000 people in North Carolina found that almost 90 percent believed in healing miracles.[10] While the sample was predominantly Christian, belief in healing miracles was just as common in those with no religion. Half of the respondents said that they had personally witnessed a healing miracle, either their own or that of a loved one.

The study was not focused on dying patients, but the findings may have implications for patients dealing with end-of-life decisions. Belief in healing miracles may partially explain why some patients and families are hopeful of healing even in the face of a very poor prognosis. While such a hopeful outlook could facilitate discussion of end-of-life decisions such as resuscitation status, as in the study of HIV patients,[2] an irrational belief in miracle healing could impede appropriate decision making. Patients and families could come into conflict with medical and nursing staff who have a more pragmatic outlook based on the scientific prognosis. Greater understanding and appreciation of the patient's spiritual belief in healing miracles could help reduce such conflict.

A belief in an afterlife is a prominent part of many faith traditions. Belief in heaven and hell has become a part of the culture in

U.S. society. Even Hollywood films have attempted to depict what existence would be like in the afterlife *(Ghost, What Dreams May Come,* among others). The Christian faith tradition holds that the person's eternal destiny is decided on the basis of beliefs or actions during this lifetime. This faith tradition may provoke great anxiety in some who are terminally ill and facing an uncertain future. "Dying when removed or cut off from God or a higher power" and "Not being forgiven by God" are two of the top three spiritual worries people have when they think about their own death (see Table 9.1).[1] Patients may feel that they have certain tasks they need to perform or have issues they need to resolve, but may not have the strength or mobility to accomplish these functions. Failure to resolve these issues can lead to anxiety, fear, and guilt. From the point of view of many patients, such unresolved issues could have eternal consequences, and are understandably related to fear of death and death anxiety. Finding out whether patients view the afterlife as a comforting or threatening place may provide insight into patients' anxieties as they face death.

SUMMARY

Spiritual issues are among the most important issues facing patients, and may play a role in patients' fears, anxieties, and willingness to discuss end-of-life issues. Physicians should recognize the role of spirituality in dying patients and inquire about spiritual needs and concerns in such patients. Patients' beliefs about the forgiveness of God, the afterlife, and healing miracles are related to patients' views of death and their preparation for it. Physicians should be sensitive to patients' individual beliefs, and refer patients for spiritual counseling when appropriate.

QUESTIONS FOR DISCUSSION

1. Have you or a physician with whom you have worked addressed spiritual issues in the context of end-of-life decisions? Were the patients' spiritual beliefs a help or a hindrance in addressing end-of-life decisions?

2. How could you open a discussion about spiritual beliefs with a dying patient? What issues would you address?
3. What experience have you had with spirituality as a coping mechanism in dying patients? Was the patient's spirituality harmful or helpful?
4. Have you ever asked a patient about belief in miracles? If not, do you think it would be helpful in understanding the patient's perspective?
5. Have you witnessed conflict between medical personnel and families regarding applying or withholding life-sustaining treatment? What was the basis of the conflict? Would a spiritual perspective be helpful in illuminating the issues?

Chapter 10

Spirituality in Special
Patient Populations: Surgical Patients

CHAPTER OBJECTIVES

1. To review the role of religion and spirituality in preparing for surgery
2. To review the importance of religious and spiritual factors in surgical recovery
3. To review how to address spiritual concerns in the surgical patient

INTRODUCTION

Patients undergoing a major surgical procedure often report feeling helpless, fearful, and vulnerable. The stress of an upcoming operation is felt by family members as well as by the patient having the procedure. Preparing for surgery helps patients and families deal with surgery and reduce the attendant anxiety and fear. The spirituality of patients plays a role in preparing for surgery, coping with the sudden need for surgery, and coping after a surgical procedure.

BEFORE SURGERY

Religious commitment helps many patients deal with the stress of upcoming surgery. Studies document higher self-esteem and diminished anxiety and depression in patients who participate regularly in religious activities.[1,2] Bernie Siegel, MD, in *Love, Medi-*

cine, and Miracles documents dozens of cases in which allowing patients to use their own spiritual strength enabled them to manage their experience with surgery in a more positive way. A positive attitude, whether on the basis of daily meditation, prayer, or faith in God, helps patients prepare for surgery (see Case 10.1).

SURGERY AND PRAYER

Prayer is one of the most commonly used spiritual resources in the surgical setting. Surveys of patients confirm frequent use of prayer in response to acute medical illness.[3-5] One study reported on the use of prayer by 100 patients about to undergo cardiac surgery.[6] Ninety-six percent reported using prayer to deal with the

---

Case 10.1

Nelson was a fifty-six-year-old man with a loving and supportive wife, and a twelve-year-old child. He had symptoms of abdominal pain and bloating, and went to see his family doctor. Subsequent tests showed that he had colon cancer. He was referred to a general surgeon, who recommended surgery and placement of a colostomy.

Nelson and his family were in shock emotionally; this vital and energetic husband and father was now facing the challenge of major surgery. Nelson was anxious and frightened, but did not feel helpless. He and his family were very religious, and spiritually connected with their congregation. Church members prayed for Nelson corporately as well as individually. Prayer lists and telephone prayer chains were activated. Despite his fear and anxiety, Nelson approached the upcoming surgery with quiet confidence. He felt his own prayers were bolstered by those of his congregation. He had confidence in his surgeon, as well as other medical professionals who were involved. When asked the reason for his calm demeanor and quiet confidence that things would go well, he replied that God was supplying him with strength.

Questions for Discussion

1. What was Nelson's reaction to his diagnosis and planned surgery?
2. What spiritual resources did Nelson use? What other resources have you observed patients using to prepare for surgery?
3. Does the health team need to be aware of the patient's coping strategy? Why or why not?

stress of surgery, and 70 percent gave prayer the highest possible rating for helpfulness.

Prayer is often an important medium for relieving the burden, anxiety, and stress of upcoming surgery. Patients often request prayer by the chaplain or others, despite their own ability to pray for themselves. Many religious faiths have pastoral prayer as a common tradition.

Prayer also may benefit patients' surgical recovery as well as their attitudes. In one study, patients who frequently prayed to God had less trouble following the prescribed medical regimen than others.[2] In another study, those who prayed with chaplains had one-third less use of pain medication in the hospital postoperative period.[7]

RELIGIOUS/SPIRITUAL FACTORS AND SURGICAL RECOVERY

Religious beliefs and practices have been linked to improved survival in surgical patients. In a study of 232 patients undergoing elective heart surgery, the death rate of patients six months after surgery was significantly lower among churchgoers than nonchurchgoers (5 percent versus 12 percent), particularly among those who found significant strength and comfort in religious beliefs and practices.[8] Those with low social support and low religiousness were twelve times more likely to die than those with strong levels of social support and religiousness. Even after controlling for social confounders, those with high religiousness were three times less likely to die after surgery than nonreligious patients.[8] Other research studies have found improved ambulation after hip surgery[1] and improved overall functioning twelve months after cardiac surgery[2] among more religious patients. The implication of this data is that being nonreligious is a risk factor for poorer surgical outcome.

ADDRESSING SPIRITUAL CONCERNS AND MOBILIZING SPIRITUAL RESOURCES IN THE SURGICAL PATIENT

Research suggests that addressing spiritual concerns in the surgical patient may reduce preoperative anxiety and reduce postoperative pain.[6,7] One simple strategy is to take a spiritual history, listen to any spiritual concerns, and refer the patient for spiritual counseling if needed.

First, assess the patient's spirituality, determining preexisting spiritual support and resources (see Chapter 6). By showing sensitivity and concern for the patients' spiritual side, clinicians give patients the opportunity to mobilize their own spiritual resources, and grant legitimacy to their use. Almost all patients feel their spiritual health is as important as their physical health, and most want physicians to address their spiritual awareness. Next, listen for any specific spiritual concerns, and gently inquire about spiritual support. Then refer the patient to the chaplain or other qualified spiritual counselor, especially patients undergoing cancer surgery or other major surgery. Use of chaplain services can reduce length of stay in surgical patients (Chapter 8), reduce use of pain medications, and activate spiritual resources associated with improved postoperative functioning and mortality. Some surgeons may feel comfortable in participating in patient-led prayers.

Patients undergoing surgery may feel singled out by God for stress or punishment. Patients may ask "why me?" or "why now?" when faced with an acute illness or injury requiring surgery. Such questions transcend the accepted boundaries of social support, and are not answered by more family, friends, or finances. Such questions also may be beyond the skills and time available for surgeons to address them directly, but surgeons can play an important role by opening a dialogue about spiritual issues and being supportive of spiritual care (see Figure 10.1).

The chaplain can often spend extended time with the patient to address spiritual questions and mobilize the patients' inner resources. The chaplain also may be the prayer leader for family and friends visiting the patient. Surgeons can initiate the spiritual care process by taking a spiritual history and listening to the patient's concerns.

SUMMARY

Religion and spirituality play an important role in assisting patients to prepare for surgery. Patients often use prayer and meditation to cope with the stress and anxiety of undergoing a surgical procedure. A few

FIGURE 10.1. Interview with Mohammed R. Alijani, MD, FACS

Dr. Alijani is Professor of Surgery and Director of Kidney and Pancreas Transplantation at Georgetown University Medical Center. Dr. Alijani received a surgical transplant fellowship at the University of Iowa and served at the Walter Reed Army Hospital and the National Naval Medical Center before joining the faculty at Georgetown in 1980. A practicing Muslim, Dr. Alijani immigrated to the United States from Iran in 1971.

As an experienced surgeon, what role have you seen religion play in health, specifically surgery?

I have no doubt in my mind that faith plays a major role in our normal daily life as well as when any stress occurs. I have seen it in so many patients and in my own life. Handling stress if you do have faith is much easier than if you don't. Most people are scared when they find out they have to have surgery. In major surgery, you have to be mentally prepared. Some patients are in denial. They don't accept dialysis or surgery. Patients with faith are different. My observation is those who have faith listen to you carefully, trust you, and are very cooperative in terms of evaluation. It's a lot of work to prepare a patient for activati[on] onto a transplant list. Those who have faith place their trust in the surgeon and expedite the process. After surgery they say, "I trust you and I have faith. You do what you think is appropriate. You treat me and God cures me." Most of these people do better. They recover better. Religious patients tend to comply better—they keep appointments; they take their medications.

[Can you] give me an example of the role of faith in a patient's life from your practice of surgery?

I had one patient whose kidney I had to remove due to renal-cell carcinoma. One year later, a sonogram revealed a cancerous lesion in the other kidney. I had to remove that kidney as well, leaving him with no kidneys. After a year of dialysis, he received a kidney transplant. He is now doing extremely well. From beginning to end, the man showed his faith. He said, "Do whatever is appropriate—I trust you." In contrast, I had another patient who also had a kidney transplant due to renal-cell carcinoma, but six months later he expired. He had no faith. He cried like a little boy. He gave up. His immune system gave up. I have seen many of these examples in my practice since 1965, particularly in the last twenty years.

As a practicing Muslim, you fast during the month of Ramadan. How does that affect your abilities to perform surgery?

Hypoglycemia impacts our performance as surgeons causing our stamina and the stability of our hands to decline. Therefore, we try to eat some-

FIGURE 10.1 *(continued)*

---

thing before a long surgery and stay away from drinking coffee. I have thirty days of Ramadan, one month every year. I have never missed a day of fasting. I wake at 4:00 a.m., I pray, and I don't eat anything. I go until 6:30 p.m. before I eat. It is amazing that on those days I have never felt that I had to have lunch. Mentally, I was prepared and I didn't see any impact on my surgical performance. But if I have to fast on a day that is not Ramadan, I see the impact in my performance without question. During the month of Ramadan, I don't have any such problem.

How do you address spiritual issues as you interact with your patients?

Until the last two or three years I shied away from this. I thought that I should not be the one to bring spiritual issues up. By listening to the patients, I would often know who had faith and who didn't, but we might go on without bringing up the issue. However, recently I began to change. Now, I don't mind raising the issue first. We must be very delicate and careful to not hurt patients' feelings. I am Muslim but I believe in Jesus since we have respect for all of the prophets. I am respectful of all religious people, and when we do talk about faith, they know I practice my own religion. What we have in common is God.

Source: Matthews, D.A., Ed. Interview with Mohammed R. Alijani, MD, FACS. *Faith and Medicine Connection,* 1998; 2(3):4. Reprinted with permission.

studies have shown a reduction in anxiety and postoperative pain among patients who use prayer and other religious practices. Surgeons can facilitate spiritual care by taking a spiritual history, listening to patients' concerns, and routinely referring patients to chaplains for counseling.

QUESTION FOR DISCUSSION

1. What spiritual concerns does facing surgery reveal? How can clinicians assist patients in addressing such concerns?

Chapter 11

Integrating Spirituality
into Clinical Practice

CHAPTER OBJECTIVES

1. To understand the spectrum of involvement of health professionals in spirituality
2. To understand the skills and attitudes needed to effectively integrate spirituality into practice
3. To review the importance of including spirituality in the education of health professionals

INTRODUCTION

Effectively integrating spirituality into clinical practice involves an understanding of the possible levels of involvement, as well as acquiring certain clinical skills and attitudes. Several barriers have prevented the routine incorporation of spirituality into medical care, including the mind-body perspective that excludes spiritual factors and related considerations from clinical skills. The preceding chapters have discussed the rationale for adding spirituality to the biopsychosocial model and have provided information to enhance knowledge and clinical care. Patients' religious and spiritual beliefs have been found to affect perception of illness (Chapter 3), health outcomes, including mortality (Chapter 4), and decision making about care at the end of life (Chapter 9). Several methods of taking a spiritual history have been presented (Chapter 6), and ethical aspects of spiritual involvement have been considered (Chapter 7). The goal of this chapter is to assist the learner in overcoming the barriers to the integration of spirituality into clinical practice.

SPECTRUM OF INVOLVEMENT

The concept of a spectrum of involvement represents the idea that different practitioners will be involved in patients' spirituality to different degrees. At one end of the "spectrum" is the minimal level of involvement (Level I) of taking a spiritual history and referring patients to chaplains (Level II) (see Figure 11.1).

At the other end of the spectrum are the more intimate activities of praying with patients and doing spiritual counseling (Levels III and IV). Levels I and II are appropriate for all physicians and other health professionals and assure the delivery of spiritually competent care. Taking a spiritual history and referring patients for counseling regarding spiritual concerns should be integrated into clinical practice as a part of routine medical care. Levels III and IV activities involve spiritual intervention that may be meaningful to many physicians and patients, but may be appropriate in fewer situations or for physicians who have particular interest, experience, or training.

It is the goal of this text to equip all health professionals with the basic knowledge and skills necessary to take a spiritual history from a patient. The ability to perform an assessment of a patient's spiritual and religious beliefs as they relate to health is a basic clinical skill that can be mastered by all physicians, as well as many other health professionals. Because patients' religious views touch many areas of medical care, including attitudes toward abortion, contraception, euthanasia, blood transfusions, organ transplants, and many other areas of consequence, all physicians need to be comfortable obtaining patients' views of pertinent medical issues. Identifying patients with spiritual concerns and referring such patients to a certified chaplain or other ministerial counselor should be routine in medical

FIGURE 11.1. Spectrum of Involvement in Spirituality

Level I	II	III	IV
All		Few	
Taking a spiritual history and referral to chaplain	Spiritual counseling in collaboration with chaplain	Praying with patients/counseling those of the same faith	Counseling patients of different faiths

practice.[1] All health professionals should be trained to collaborate regarding medical and spiritual issues (Chapter 8).

Level II involvement is characterized by counseling patients who have spiritual concerns. Ethical issues are more prevalent at this level, and respect for patient autonomy and privacy must be maintained. Nevertheless, through training or experience, many physicians are qualified to counsel patients regarding medical decision making that involves a conflict with spiritual or religious values such as blood transfusion or terminal care issues. Many physicians already counsel patients about such medical issues, but without benefit of an understanding of the religious and spiritual conflicts the patient is facing. Appropriate spiritual clinical skills training will improve doctor-patient interaction in situations in which spiritual issues currently are neglected.

Level III involvement adds the element of participation in prayer with patients. Praying with patients is one of the most intimate forms of spiritual interaction in practice.[2] Although the first two levels characterize the spiritually competent physician, Level III involvement is not required for clinically competent care. Participating in patients' prayers can be especially meaningful and rewarding,[3] but can also be uncomfortable in situations when the faith traditions of the physician and patient are incongruent. Forty-eight percent of patients in one study wanted their physicians to pray with them;[4] however, the study did not investigate whether patients were comfortable when the physician's religious tradition was different from their own. Some physicians already pray with patients and participate in spiritual and worship activities together as members of the same religious congregation outside of the medical office.[2,3]

Level IV involvement is the deepest level of spiritual involvement. Physicians with special training, such as theological degrees or unique clinical experience, may elect to include direct spiritual counseling as part of their practice. This could include practices at religious hospitals that have a homogenous population, mission hospitals that openly combine medical and spiritual care, and certain outpatient clinics and practices. Counseling patients of various religious and spiritual backgrounds regarding their spiritual concerns falls within the field of pastoral care and is best handled by certified chaplains. Physicians cannot replace chaplains; the two roles are distinct.[5]

Effectively integrating spirituality into practice is a challenge for modern medicine.[6] Clinicians are immediately faced with the conflict of treating patients who are, as a group, mostly religious, in a largely secular medical system. Most physicians practice in a pluralistic environment, treating patients of various ethnic, cultural, and religious backgrounds. Physicians themselves may have strong religious or spiritual beliefs that affect their motivation to practice, their outlook, and their view of the medical decisions facing their patients. They must practice their profession knowing that no one can be totally unbiased in his or her human interactions. Being sensitive to patients' religious and spiritual beliefs while holding on to their own, they must listen to their patients' spiritual concerns and deal with them in the context of professional medical care. Can it be done? It is the premise of this text that it can be done, with appropriate training and sensitivity. The following excerpt gives an example of one practicing physician's approach:

> . . . I would like to offer one approach to integrating the issue of faith and illness into daily practice. I regularly explore the impact of my patients' faith experience on their health, particularly during times of illness and adjustment. I introduce the subject by asking, "Do you belong to any particular church or subscribe to a particular faith?" If they respond affirmatively, I ask what impact their illness has had on their faith and whether their faith experience has been helpful in coping with their illness. I also ask if they have spoken to anyone about this, particularly their minister, and what effect that has had.
>
> If they report that they currently have no particular allegiance to any faith, I ask about their past experiences. Past faith experiences are often, in part, the foundation of their current beliefs, which they rely on to cope with difficulties. On occasion, an unsettled conflict about their past religious experience is uncovered. When this occurs, it is helpful to refer patients to their spiritual advisor for resolution of the conflict. This may open the door to spiritual support through their difficult times.

As for the faith experience of the physicians, once the subject has been broached, patients often inquire of the physician's experience. When they find it to be common with theirs, it often gives them comfort. Patients often find comfort in knowing that their physician prays about his or her work and for the patients. Occasionally, patients have requested that I pray for them and, and less often, with them.

If we share different experiences, then a comment that reflects the physician's understanding of some common ground is usually helpful. If the physician is totally unfamiliar with the patient's faith experience, then a request that the patient explain the basic tenets of that faith will usually foster a helpful understanding. Finally, asking if the patient would like to be remembered in the physician's daily prayer avoids the pitfall of the patient who does not want this and also conveys a clear message of the physician's respect for the patient and the patient's autonomy.

Given the increasing awareness of the impact of the faith experience on illness and health, a working approach to addressing this aspect of our patients' life experiences is needed. I have outlined an approach that has been successful in my practice. More work needs to be done to identify methods with proven benefits that physicians can comfortably apply to their practices. (Lijoi, A.F. Reprinted with permission from the *Journal of Family Practice* 45(1):15, 1997).

INTEGRATING SPIRITUALITY INTO HEALTH PROFESSIONS EDUCATION

Through experience and training, physicians can become more skilled at spiritual assessment and referral, and become more comfortable with addressing patients' spiritual needs. Better medical school education, residency training, and continuing medical education will equip future physicians with the tools to integrate spirituality into clinical practice.

Patients desire caring and compassionate physicians who offer humane concern for them. Integral to incorporating this humane concern into care is training to enhance physicians' receptivity to patients who want to talk about the spirituality that gives meaning to their lives.[7] A growing number of medical schools offer courses on religious and spiritual issues.[8] Study of religion and spirituality can be a framework for learning person-centered medicine and an appreciation for human diversity.[9]

A curriculum in spirituality and medicine should include the following components:[8,9]

1. The importance of religion and spirituality in the lives of patients
2. Patients' religion/spirituality as both a challenge and a resource for the patient and the physician
3. How to take a spiritual history as a routine part of medical assessment
4. Review of the empirical literature regarding religion, spirituality, and health
5. Importance of including chaplains as a part of collaborative care in the health care team
6. Integrating religious/spiritual issues into problem-based learning
7. Ethical issues in spiritual involvement
8. The role of spiritual issues in patients facing major surgery and the end of life

Students should also be encouraged to explore their own beliefs and consider how those beliefs affect their care of patients. The American Association of Medical Colleges (AAMC) has conducted conferences regarding spirituality in the curriculum.

Training in spiritual clinical skills and spiritual issues in health should continue in residency. Spiritual training is being included in some psychiatry[10] and family medicine[11] residencies, and perhaps others. The goals of the curriculum in residency are to provide training in spiritual assessment, referral, and collaboration, and gain supervised clinical experience dealing with patients' spiritual concerns.

Continuing education for practicing physicians, medical school faculty, and residency program faculty should expand to provide training in spirituality that most likely was not available during their medical school or residency training. Courses such as the one sponsored by Harvard Medical School ("Spirituality and Healing in

Medicine") can help physicians address patients' spiritual concerns and acquire the skills to teach future medical students and residents.

SUMMARY

Awareness of the spiritual aspects of medical care can expand and enrich medical practice. Physicians and other health professionals can be involved in patients' spirituality at various levels. The spectrum of involvement ranges from spiritual assessment and referral (Level I, II) to praying with patients and counseling them (Level III, IV). The spiritually competent clinician needs to master the first two levels. Effectively integrating spirituality into practice is a challenge that can be met through training that enables students to acquire sensitivity and appreciation for patients' spiritual and religious beliefs. Training should continue in residency and beyond so that health professionals can meet the spiritual health needs of patients.

Notes

Chapter 1

1. Dougherty WJ, Baird MA, Becker LA. Family medicine and the biopsychosocial model. *Advances* 1986; 3:17-18.

2. Medalie JH. Angina pectoris: A validation of the biopsychosocial model. *Journal of Family Practice* 1990; 30(3)3:273-280.

3. Dossey L. *Healing words.* San Francisco. Harper, 1993.

4. Larson DB, Milano MAG. Are religion and spirituality clinically relevant in health care? *Mind/Body Medicine* 1995; 1(3):147-157.

5. Craigie FC, Larson DB, Liu I. References to religion in the *Journal of Family Practice:* Dimensions and valence of spirituality. *Journal of Family Practice* 1990; 30(4):472-480.

6. Matthews DA, Larson DB, Barry CP. *The faith factor: An annotated bibliography of clinical research on spiritual subjects.* Radnor, PA. John Templeton Foundation, 1993.

7. Levin JS. How prayer heals: A theoretical model. *Alternative Therapy in Health and Medicine* 1996; 2(1):66-73.

8. Levin JS. Religion and health: Is there an association, is it valid, and is it causal? *Social Science and Medicine* 1994; 38(11):1475-1482.

9. Weaver AJ, Flannelly LT, Flannelly KJ, Koenig HG, Larson DB. An analysis of research of religious and spiritual variables in three major health nursing journals, 1991-1995. *Issues in Mental Health Nursing,* 1998; 19(3):263-276.

10. Engel GL. Clinical application of the biopsychosocial model. In DE Reiser and DH Rosen, (Eds.). *Medicine as a human experience* (pp. 43-60). Gaithersburg, MD: Aspen Publishers, 1984.

11. Melamed BG. The neglected psychological-physical interface. *Health Psychology* 1995; 14(5):371-373.

12. Dantzer R. Stress and disease: A psychobiological perspective. *Annals of Behavioral Medicine* 1991; 13(12):205-210.

13. Engel GL. The need for a new medical model: A challenge for biomedicine. *Science* 1977; 196(4286):129-136.

14. Engel GL. The biomedical model: A Procrustean bed? *Man and Medicine* 1979; 4(4):257-275.

15. Friedman M, Rosenman RH. *Type A behavior and your heart.* New York: Alfred A. Knopf, 1974.

16. Frasure-Smith N, Lesperance F, Talajic M. The impact of negative emotions on prognosis following myocardial infarction: Is it more than depression? *Health Psychology* 1995; 14(5):388-398.

17. Greer S, Morris T, Pettingale KW. Psychological response to breast cancer: Effects on outcome. *Lancet* 1979; 2(8146):785-787.

18. Schleifer SJ, Keller SE, Camerino M, Thornton JC, Stein M. Suppression of lymphocyte stimulation following bereavement. *JAMA* 1983; 250(3):374-377.

19. Cohen S, Rodriquez MS. Pathways linking affective disturbance and physical disorders. *Health Psychology* 1995; 14(5):374-380.

20. McWhinney I. Time, change and the physician. Plenary address to the Society of Teachers of Family Medicine, 16th Annual Spring Conference, Boston, Massachusetts. May 1983.

21. King DE, Hueston W, Rudy M. Religious affiliation and obstetric outcome. *Southern Medical Journal* 1994; 87(11):1125-1128.

22. Koenig HG, Cohen MJ, Blazer DG, Pieper C, Meador KG, Shelp F, Goli V, Dipasquale B. Religious coping and depression among elderly hospitalized medically ill men. *American Journal of Psychiatry* 1992; 149(12):1693-1700.

23. Larson DB, Sherrill KA, Lyons JS, Craigie FC Jr, Thielman SB, Greenwold MA. Associations between dimensions of religious commitment and mental health reported in the *American Journal of Psychiatry* and *Archives of General Psychiatry:* 1978-1989. *American Journal of Psychiatry* 1992; 149(4):557-559.

24. Idler EL, Kasl SV. Religion, disability, depression, and the timing of death. *American Journal of Sociology* 1992; 97(4):1052-1079.

25. Oman D, Reed D. Religion and morality in the community-dwelling elderly. *American Journal of Public Health* 1998; 88(10):1469-1475.

26. Pressman P, Lyons JS, Larson DB, Strain JJ. Religious belief, depression, and ambulation status in elderly women with broken hips. *American Journal of Psychiatry* 1990; 147(6):758-760.

27. Kendler KS, Gardner CO, Prescott CA. Religion, psychopathology, and substance use and abuse: A multimeasure, genetic-epidemiologic study. *American Journal of Psychiatry* 1997; 154(3):322-329.

28. Levin JS, Markides JS, Ray LA. Religious attendance and psychological well-being in Mexican Americans: A panel analysis of three-generation data. *Gerontologist* 1996; 36(4):454-463.

29. Okun MA, Stock WA, Haring MJ, Witter RA. Health and subjective well-being: A meta-analysis. *International Journal of Aging and Human Development,* 1984; 19(2): 111-132.

30. Benson P. Religion and substance use. In JF Schumaker (ed.) *Religion and mental health.* New York: Oxford University Press, 1992.

31. Schwab R, Petersen KU. Religiousness: Its relation to loneliness, neuroticism, and subjective well-being. *Journal of the Scientific Study of Religion* 1990; 29(3):335-345.

32. Gorsuch RL. Religious aspects of substance abuse and recovery. *Journal of Social Issues* 1995; 51(2):65-83.

33. Payne IR, Bergin AE, Bielema KA, Jenkins PH. Review of religion and mental health: Prevention and enhancement of psychosocial functioning. *Prevention in Human Services,* 1991; 9(2):11-40.

34. Donahue MJ. Intrinsic and extrinsic religiousness: Review and meta-analysis. *Journal of Personality and Social Psychology,* 1985; 48(2):400-419.

35. Troyer H. Review of cancer among four religious sects: Evidence that lifestyles are distinctive sets of risk factors. *Social Science and Medicine* 1988; 26(10):1007-1017.

36. Jarvis GK, Northcutt HC. Religion and differences in morbidity and mortality. *Social Science and Medicine* 1987; 25(7):813-824.

37. Scotch NA. Sociocultural factors in the epidemiology of Zulu hypertension. *American Journal of Public Health* 1963; 53(August):1205-1213.

38. Scotch NA. A preliminary report on the relation of sociocultural factors to hypertension among the Zulu. *Annals of New York Academy of Science* 1960; 84(December 8):1000-1009.

39. Friedlander Y, Kark JD. Familial aggregation of blood pressure in a Jewish population sample in Jerusalem among ethnic and religious groups. *Social Biology* 1984; 31(1-2):75-90.

40. Walsh A. The prophylactic effect of religion on blood pressure levels among samples of immigrants. *Social Science and Medicine* 1980; 14B(1):59-63.

41. Walsh A, Walsh PA. Social support, assimilation and biological effect blood pressure levels. *Internal Migration Revue* 1987; 21(3):577-591.

42. Graham TW, Kaplan BH, Cornoni-Huntley JC, James SA, Becker C, Hames CG, Heyden S. Frequency of church attendance and blood pressure elevation. *Journal of Behavioral Medicine* 1978; 1(1):37-43.

43. Levin JS, Markides KS. Religion and health in Mexican-Americans. *Journal of Religion and Health* 1985; 24(1):60-69.

44. Hutchinson J. Association between stress and blood pressure variation in a Caribbean population. *American Journal of Physical Anthropology* 1986; 71(1):69-79.

45. Larson DB, Koenig HG, Kaplan BH, Greenberg RS, Logue E, Tyroler H. The impact of religion of men's blood pressure. *Journal of Religion and Health* 1989; 28(4):265-278.

46. Koenig HG, Cohen HJ, Hays JC, Larson DB, Blazer DG. Attendance at religious services, interleukin-6, and other biological parameters of immune function in older adults. *International Journal of Psychiatric Medicine* 1997; 27(3):233-250.

47. Koenig HG, Beacon LB, Dayringer R. Physician perspectives on the role of religion in the physician-older patient relationship. *Journal of Family Practice* 1989; 28:(4)441-448.

48. Mansfield C, Mitchell J, King DE. The doctor as God's mechanic? Beliefs of a southeastern rural population. Presented at the annual meeting of the North American Primary Care Research Group, November 14, 1997, Orlando, Florida.

49. Moyers PA. Occupational meanings and spirituality: The quest for sobriety. *American Journal of Occupational Therapy* 1997; 51(3):207-214.

50. Watson CG, Hancock M, Gearhart LP, Mendez CM, Malovrh P, Raden M. A comparative outcome study of frequency, moderate, occasional, and nonattenders of Alcoholics Anonymous. *Journal of Clinical Psychology* 1997; 53(3):209-214.

51. Byrd RC. Positive therapeutic effects of intercessory prayer in a coronary care unit population. *Southern Medical Journal* 1988; 81(7):836-839.

52. Sicher F, Targ E, Moore D, Smith HS. A randomized double-blind study of the effect of distant healing in a population with advanced AIDS. Report of a small scale study. *Western Journal of Medicine* 1998; 169(6):356-363.

53. King DE, Bushwick B. Beliefs and attitudes of hospital inpatients about faith healing and prayer. *Journal of Family Practice* 1994; 39(4):349-352.

54. Maugans TA, Wadland WC. Religion and family medicine: A survey of physicians and patients. *Journal of Family Practice* 1991; 32(2):210-213.

55. Melone L, Hall L. Patients seek acknowledgement, incorporation of their spirituality in medical treatment. Internet: <http://www.templeton.org/course98/pressrelease12_14.asp>; June 18, 1999.

56. Fitchett G, Burton LA, Sivan AB. The religious needs and resources of psychiatric inpatients. *Journal of Nervous and Mental Diseases* 1997; 185(5): 320-326.

57. McBride JL, Arthur G, Brooks R, Pilkington L. The relationship between a patient's spirituality and health experiences. *Family Medicine* 1998; 30(2):122-126.

58. Sharp CG. Use of chaplaincy in the neonatal intensive care unit. *Southern Medical Journal* 1991; 84(12):1482-1486.

59. Anderson JM, Anderson LJ, Felsenthal G. Pastoral needs and support within an inpatient rehabilitation unit. *Archives of Physical Medicine and Rehabilitation* 1993; 74(6):574-578.

Chapter 2

1. The Gallup Poll. Public Opinion 1997. Scholarly Resources, Inc. Wilmington, Delaware; 1998.

2. Gallup G. Religion at home and abroad. *Public Opinion* 1979; March-May:38-39.

3. Gallup G. *Religion in America 1990.* The Princeton Religion Research Center, Princeton, NJ; 1990.

4. Barry A. Kosmin and Seymour P. Lachman. *One nation under God.* New York, New York; Harmony Books, 1993.

5. Koenig HG. Religious attitudes and practices of hospitalized medically ill older adults. *International Journal of Geratric Psychiatry* 1998; 13(4):213-224.

6. King DE, Bushwick B. Beliefs and attitudes of hospital inpatients about faith healing and prayer. *Journal of Family Practice* 1994; 39(4):349-352.

7. Manning KM. A Catholic viewpoint. *Australian Family Physician* 1986; 15(4):493-497.

8. Fellows, WJ. *Religious east and west.* New York. Holt, Rinehart and Winston, 1979.

9. Ewers GA. Four viewpoints: Churches of Christ. *Australian Family Physician* 1986; 15(8):1024.

10. Levi JS. Jewish medical ethics. *Australian Family Physician* 1986; 15(1): 17-19.

11. Khan SN. The Islamic viewpoint. *Australian Family Physician* 1986; 15(2):179-180.

12. MacLean D. Jehovah's Witnesses. *Australian Family Physician* 1986; 15(6):772-774.

13. Oats WN. Four viewpoints: The Religious Society of Friends (Quakers). *Australian Family Physician* 1986; 15(8):1025.

Chapter 3

1. Maugans TA. The SPIRITual history. *Archives of Family Medicine* 1996; 5(1):11-16.

2. McBride JL, Arthur G, Brooks R, Pilkington L. The relationship between patient's spirituality and health experiences. *Family Medicine* 1998; 30(2):122-126.

3. Hill PC, Butler EM. The role of religion in promoting physical health. *Journal of Psychology and Christianity* 1995; 14(2):141-155.

4. King DE, Bushwick B. Beliefs and attitudes of hospital inpatients about faith healing and prayer. *Journal of Family Practice* 1994; 39(4):349-352.

5. Maugans TA, Wadland WC. Religion and family medicine: A survey of physicians and patients. *Journal of Family Practice* 1991; 32(2):210-213.

6. McNichol T. The new faith in medicine. *USA Weekend* 1996; April 5-7: 4-5.

7. King DE, Sobal J, DeForge BR. Family practice patients' experiences and beliefs in faith healing. *Journal of Family Practice* 1988; 27(5):505-508.

8. Matthews DA, McCullough ME, Larson DB, Koenig HG, Swyers JP, Milano MG. Religious commitment and health status. *Archives of Family Medicine* 1998; 7(2):118-124.

9. Koenig HG, Kvale JN, Ferrel C. Religion and well-being in later life. *The Gerentologist* 1988; 28(1):18-28.

10. Kass JD, Friedman R, Lesermann J, Zuttermeister PC, Benson H. Health outcomes and a new index of spiritual experience. *Journal of the Scientific Study of Religion* 1991; 30(2):203-211.

11. Nelsen EC, Landgraft JM, Hays RD, Wassen JH, Kirk JW. The functional status of patients: How can it be measured in physicians' offices? *Medical Care* 1990; 28(12):1111-1126.

12. Koenig HG, Moberg DO, Kvale J. Religious activities and attitudes of older adults in a geriatric assessment clinic. *Journal of American Geriatric Society* 1988; 36(4):362-374.

13. Byrd RC. Positive therapeutic effects of intercessory prayer in a coronary care unit population. *Southern Medical Journal* 1988; 81(7): 826-829.

14. Dossey L. *Healing words: The power of prayer and the practice of medicine.* San Francisco, CA: Harper San Francisco, 1993.

15. Duckro PN, Magaletta PR. The effect of prayer on physical health: Experimental evidence. *Journal of Religion and Health* 1994; 33(3):211-219.

16. McCullough ME. Prayer and health: Conceptual issues, research review, and research agenda. *Journal of Psychology and Theology* 1995; 23(1):15-29.

17. Magaletta PR, Duckro PN, Staten SF. Prayer in office practice: On the threshold of integration. *Journal of Family Practice* 1997; 44(3):254-256.

18. Sloan RP, Bagiella E, Powell T. Religion, spirituality, and medicine. *Lancet* 1999; 353(9153):664-667.

19. Waldfogel S. Spirituality in medicine. *Primary Care* 1997; 24(4):963-976.

20. Benson H. *Timeless healing.* New York: Scribner and Sons, 1996.

Chapter 4

1. Levin JS. Religion and health: Is there an association, is it valid, and is it causal? *Social Science and Medicine* 1994; 38(11):1475-1482.

2. Craigie FC, Larson DB, Liu IY. References to religion in the *Journal of Family Practice. Journal of Family Practice* 1990; 30(4):477-480.

3. Levin JS, Schiller PL. Is there a religious factor in health? *Journal of Religion and Health* 1987; 26(1):9-36.

4. Matthews DA, McCullough ME, Larson DB, Koenig HG, Sawyers JP, Milano MG. Religious commitment and health status. *Archives of Family Medicine* 1998; 7(2):118-124.

5. Koenig HG, Cohen HJ, Blazer DG, Pieper C, Meador KG, Shelp F, Goli V, Dipasquale B. Religious coping and depression among elderly, hospitalized, medically ill men. *American Journal of Psychiatry* 1992; 149(12):1693-1700.

6. Park C, Cohen LH, Herb L. Intrinsic religiousness and religious coping as life stress moderators for Catholics versus Protestants. *Journal of Personality and Social Psychology* 1990; 59(3):562-574.

7. Fallot RD (Ed.). *Spirituality and religion in recovery from mental illness.* San Francisco: Jossey-Bass, Inc., 1998.

8. King DE, Sobal J, Deforge BR. Family practice patients' experiences and beliefs in faith healing. *Journal of Family Practice* 1988; 27:505-508.

9. King DE, Bushwick B. Beliefs and attitudes of hospital inpatients about faith healing and prayer. *Journal of Family Practice* 1994; 39(4); 349-352.

10. Williams DR, Larson DB, Buckler RE, Hechman RC, Pyle CM. Religion and psychological distress in a community sample. *Social Science and Medicine* 1991; 32(11):1257-1262.

11. Pargament KI, Ensing DS, Falgout K, Olsen B, Van Haitsma K, Warren R. God help me: Religious coping efforts as predictors of the outcomes of significant life events. *American Journal of Community Psychology* 1990; 18(11):793-824.

12. Koenig HG. *Is religion good for your health? The effects of religion on physical and mental health.* New York: The Haworth Pastoral Press; 1997.

13. Oman D, Reed D. Religion and mortality among the community-dwelling elderly. *American Journal of Public Health* 1998; 88(10):1469-1475.

14. Comstock GW, Tonaseia JA. Education and mortality in Washington County, Maryland. *Journal of Health and Social Behavior* 1978; 18(1):54-61.

15. House JS, Robbins C, Metzner HL. The association of social relationships and activities with mortality: Prospective evidence from the Tecumseh health study. *American Journal of of Epidemiology* 1982; 116(1):123-140.

16. Strawbridge WJ, Cohen RD, Shema SJ, Kaplan GA. Frequent attendance at religious services and mortality over twenty-eight years. *American Journal of of Public Health* 1997; 87(6):957-961.

17. Idler EL, Kasl SV. Religion, disability, depression, and the timing of death. *American Journal of of Sociology* 1992; 97(4):1052-1079.

18. Goldman N, Korenman S, Weinstein R. Marital status and health among the elderly. *Social Science and Medicine* 1995; 40(12):1717-1730.

19. Scotch, NA. A preliminary report on the relation of sociocultural factors to hypertension among the Zulu. *Annals of New York Academy of Science* 1960; 84(December 8):1000-1009.

20. Scotch NA. Sociocultural factors in the epidemiology of Zulu hypertension. *American Journal of Public Health* 1963; 53(August):1205-1213.

21. Friedlander Y, Kark JD. Familial aggregation of blood pressure in a Jewish population sample in Jerusalem among ethnic and religious groups. *Social Biology* 1984; 31(1-2):75-90.

22. Walsh A. The prophylactic effect of religion on blood pressure levels among a sample of immigrants. *Social Science and Medicine* 1980; 14B(1):59-63.

23. Walsh A, Walsh PA. Social support, assimilation, and biological effective blood pressure levels. *Internal Migration Revue* 1987; 21(3):577-591.

24. Graham TW, Kaplan BM, Cornoni-Huntley JC, James SA, Becker C, Hames CG, Heyden S. Frequency of church attendance and blood pressure elevation. *Journal of Behvioral Medicine* 1978; 1:37-43.

25. Levin JS, Markides KS. Religion and health in Mexican-Americans. *Journal of Religion and Health* 1985; 24(1):60-69.

26. Hutchinson J. Association between stress and blood pressure variation in a Caribbean population. *American Journal of Physical Anthropology* 1986; 71(1):69-79.

27. Larson DB, Koenig HG, Kaplan BH, Greenberg RS, Logue E, Tyroloer H. The impact of religion on men's blood pressure. *Journal of Religion and Health* 1989; 28(4):265-278.

28. Levin JS, Vanderpool HY. Is religion therapeutically significant for hypertension? *Social Science and Medicine* 1989; 29(1):69-78.

29. Koenig HG, Cohen HJ, George LK, Hays JC, Larson DB, Blazer DG. Attendance at religious services, interleukin-6, and other biological parameters of immune function in older adults. *International Journal of Psychiatry Medicine* 1997; 27(3): 233-250.

30. National Institues of Mental Health, "Facts About Depression." Internet: *www.nimh.nih.gov,* September 30, 1999.

31. Koenig HG, George LK, Peterson BL. Religiosity and remission from depression in medically ill older patients. *American Journal of Psychiatry* 1998; 155(4):536-542.

32. Propst LR, Ostrom R, Watkins P, Dean T, Mashburn D. Comparative efficacy of religious and non-religious cognitive-behavioral therapy for the treatment of clinical depression in religious individuals. *Journal of Consulting and Clinical Psychology* 1992; 60(1):94-103.

33. Johnson WB, Ridley CR. Brief Christian and non-Christian rational-emotive therapy with depressed Christian clients: An exploratory study. *Counseling and Values* 1992; 36(3):220-229.

34. Johnson WB, Devries R, Ridley CR, Pettorini D, Peterson DR. The comparative efficacy of Christian and secular rational-emotive therapy with Christian clients. *Journal of Psychology and Theology* 1994; 22(2):130-140.

Chapter 5

1. Koenig MG, Bearon LB, Hover M, Trans JL. Religious perspectives of doctors, nurses, patients, and families. *Journal of Pastoral Care* 1991; 45(3):254-267.
2. Weaver AJ, Koenig MG, Larson DB. Marriage and family therapists and the clergy: A need for collaboration, training, and research. *Journal of Marital and Family Therapy* 1997; 23(1):13-25.
3. Princeton Religious Research Center. (1996). Religion in America: Will the vitality of the church be the surprise of the 21st century? Princeton, NJ: Gallup Poll, 1996.
4. Ragan C, Malony HN, Beit-Hallahmi B. Psychologists and religion: Professional factors and personal belief. *Review of Religious Research* 1980; 21(2):208-217.
5. Bergin AE, Jensen JP. Religiosity of psychotherapists: A national survey. *Psychotherapy* 1990; 27(1): 3-7.
6. King DE, Bushwick B. Beliefs and attitudes of hospital inpatients about faith healing and prayer. *Journal of Family Practice* 1994; 39(4):349-352.
7. Ross RJ. Future of pastoral counseling: Legal and financial concerns. J. McHolland (Ed.). *In the future of pastoral counseling: Whom, how, and for what do we train?* Fairfax, VA: American Association of Pastoral Counselors. 1993.
8. Stander V, Piercy FP, MacKinnon D, Helmeke K. Spirituality, religion and family therapy: Competing or complementary worlds? *The American Journal of Family Therapy* 1994; 22(1):27-41.
9. Maugans, TA, Wadland WC. Religion and family medicine: A survey of family physicians and patients. *Journal of Family Practice* 1991; 32(2):210-213.
10. Oyama O, Koenig HG. Religious beliefs and practices in family medicine. *Archives of Family Medicine* 1998; 7(5):431-435.
11. Daaleman TP, Frey B. Spiritual and religious beliefs and practices of family physicians: A national survey. *Journal of FamilyPractice* 1999; 48(2):98-109.
12. Davis JA, Smith TW. *General Social Surveys, 1972-1985.* Chicago, IL: National Opinion Research Center, 1985.
13. American Psychiatric Association. (1975). Task Force Report 10. Psychiatrists' viewpoint on religion and their services to religious institutions and the ministry. Washington, DC, APA, 1975.
14. Ellis MR, Vinson DC, Ewigman B. Addressing spiritual concern of patients: Family physicians' attitudes and practices. *Journal of Family Practice* 1999; 48(2):105-109.
15. Olive KE. Physician religious beliefs and the physician-patient relationship: A study of devout physicians. *Southern Medical Journal* 1995; 88(12): 1249-1255.

16. King DE, Sobal J, Haggerty J, Dent M, Patton D. Experiences and attitudes about faith healing among family physicans. *Journal of Family Practice* 1992; 35(2):158-162.

17. Shafranske EP. *Religion and the clinical practice of psychology.* Washington, DC: American Psychological Association, 1996.

18. Weaver AJ, Samford JA, Kline AE, Lucas LA, Larsen DB, Koenig MG. What do psychologists know about working with the clergy? An analysis of eight APA journals: 1991-1994. *Professional Psychology: Research and Practice* 1997. 28(5):471-474.

19. Neelemen J, King MB. Psychiatrists' religious attitudes in relation to their clinical practice: A survey of 231 psychiatrists. *Acta Psychiatrica Scandinavica* 1993; 88:420-424.

20. Watters WW. *Deadly doctrine: Health, illness, and Christian God-talk.* Amherst, NY: Prometheus Books, 1992, p. 10.

21. Galanter M, Larson D, Rubenstone E. Christian psychiatry: The impact of evangelical belief on religious practice. *American Journal of Psychiatry* 1991; 148(1):90-95.

22. American Psychiatric Association Guidelines Regarding Possible Conflict Between Psychiatrists' Religious Commitment and Psychiatric Practice, 1990. Washington, DC: American Psychiatric Association.

23. Propst LR, Ostrom R, Watkins P, Dean T, Mashburn D. Comparative efficacy of religious and nonreligious cognitive-behavioral therapy for the treatment of clinical depression in religious individuals. *Journal of Consulting and Clinical Psychology* 1992; 60(1):94-103.

24. Florell JL. Crisis-intervention in orthopedic surgery: Empirical evidence of the effectivness of a chaplain working with surgery patients. *Bulletin of the American Protestant Hospital Association* 1973; 37(2):29-36.

Chapter 6

1. The Gallup Poll. Public Opinion 1997. Scholarly Resources, Inc. Wilmington, Delaware; 1998.

2. Gallup G. Religion in America 1990. The Princeton Religious Research Center, Princeton, NJ; 1990.

3. Mansfield C, Mitchell J, King DE. The doctor as God's mechanic? Beliefs of a southeastern rural population. Presented at the annual meeting of the North American Primary Care Research Group. Orlando, Florida, November 14, 1997.

4. King DE, Shende AM. Do our patients believe in miracles? Presented at the 15th WONCA World Conference. Dublin, Ireland, June 18, 1998.

5. McNichol T. The new faith in medicine. *USA Weekend* 1996; April 5-7: 4-5.

6. Fitchett G, Burton LA, Sivan AB. The religious needs and resources of psychiatric inpatients. *Journal of Nervous and Mental Disease* 1997; 185(5): 320-326.

7. Koenig HG, Cohen HJ, Blazer DG, Pieper C, Meador KG, Shelp F, Goli V, Dipasquale B. Religious coping and depression among elderly, hospitalized, medically ill men. *American Journal of Psychiatry* 1992; 149(12):1693-1700.

8. Fallot RD (Ed.). *Spirituality and religion in recovery from mental illness.* San Francisco, Jossey-Bass, Inc. 1998.

9. Koenig HG, Cohen HJ, Blazer DG, Kudler HS, Krishnan KR, Sibert TE. Religious coping and cognitive symptoms of depression in elderly medical patients. *Psychosomatics* 1995; 36(4):369-375.

10. Koenig HG, Pargament KI, Nielson J. Religious coping and health status in medically ill hospitalized older adults. *Journal of Nervous and Mental Disease* 1998; 186(9):513-521.

11. Matthews DA. Religion and spiratality in primary care. *Mind/Body Medicine* 1997; 2(1):9-19.

12. Maugans TA. The SPIRITual history. *Archives of Family Medicine* 1996; 5(1):11-16.

13. Kaldjian LC, Jekel JF, Friedland G. End-of-life decisions in HIV-positive patients: The role of spiritual beliefs. *AIDS* 1998; 12(1):103-107.

14. Roberts JA, Brown D, Elkins T, Larson DB. Factors influencing views of patients with gynecologic cancer about end-of-life decisions. *American Journal of Obstetrics and Gynecology* 1997; 176(1P+1):166-172.

15. Gibbs AW, Achterberg-Lawlis J. Spiritual values and death anxiety: Implications for counseling with terminal cancer patients. *Journal of Counseling Psychology* 1970; 25(6):563-569.

16. Yates JW, Chalmer BJ, James P, Follansee M, McKegney FP. Religion in patients with advanced cancer. *Medical and Pediatric Oncology* 1981; 9(2): 121-128.

17. Levi JS. Jewish medical ethics. *Australian Family Physician* 1986; 15(1): 17-19.

18. Zuckerman DM, Kasl SV, Ostfeld AM. Psychosocial predictors of mortality among the elderly poor. The role of religion, well-being, and social contacts. *American Journal of Epidemiology* 1984; 119(3):410-423.

19. Puchalski CM. Taking a spiritual history: FICA. *Spirituality and Medicine Connection* 1999; 3(1):1.

Chapter 7

1. Orr RD, Genecen LB. Medicine, ethics, and religion: Rational or irrational? *Journal of Medical Ethics* 1998; 24(6):385-387.

2. Thomasina DC, Loewy EH. Exploring the role of religion in medical ethics. *Cambridge Quarterly of Healthcare Ethics* 1996; 5(2):257-268.

3. Savulescu J. Two worlds apart: Religion and ethics. *Journal of Medical Ethics* 1998; 24(6):382-384.

4. Horner JS. Christian ethics—an irrelevance or the salvation of medicine? *Journal of Medical Ethics* 1994; 20(3):133-134.

5. Warshauer AD. Thoughts on the beliefs of religious and medical institutions. *North Carolina Medical Journal* 1985; 46(1):29-32.

6. Matthews DA. Religion and spirituality in primary care. *Mind/Body Medicine* 1997; 2(1):9-19.

7. Jamison JE. Spirituality and medical ethics. *American Journal of Hospice and Palliative Care* May/June 1995 12(3):41-45.

8. Wind JP. What can religion offer bioethics? *Hastings Center Report* July/August 1990:18-20.

9. Sloan RP, Bagiella E, Powell T. Religion, spirituality, and medicine. *Lancet* 1999; 353(9153):664-667.

10. Maugans TA, Wadland WC. Religion and family medicine: A survey of physicians and patients. *Journal of Family Practice* 1991, 32(2):210-212.

11. Davis DS. It ain't necessarily so: Clinicians, bioethics, and religious studies. *Journal of Clinical Ethics* 1994; 5(4):315-319.

12. Thiel MM, Robinson MR. Physicians' collaboration with chaplains: Difficulties and benefits. *Journal of Clinical Ethics,* Spring 1997; 8(1):94-103.

13. King DE, Bushwick B. Beliefs and attitudes of hospital inpatients about faith healing and prayer. *Journal of Family Practice* 1994; 39(4):349-352.

14. Bliss JR, McSherry E, Fassett J. Chaplain intervention reduces costs in major DRGs: An experimental study. In Heffernan H, McSherry E, Fitrzgerald R. (Eds). *Proceedings, NIH Clinical Center Conference on Spirituality and Health Care Outcomes,* March 21, 1995.

15. Florell JL. Crisis-intervention in orthopedic surgery: Empirical evidence of the effectiveness of a chaplain working with surgery patients. *Bulletin of the American Protestant Hospital Association* 1973; 37(2):29-36.

16. Saudia TL, Kinnery MR, Brown KC, Young-Ward L. Health locus of control and helpfulness of prayer. *Heart and Lung* 1991; 20(1):60-65.

17. Ellis MR, Vinson DC, Ewigman B. Addressing spiritual concerns of patients—family physicians' attitudes and practices. *Journal of Family Practice* 1999; 48(2):105-109.

18. Maugans TA. The SPIRITual history. *Archives of Family Medicine* 1996; 5(1):11-16.

19. Wood DK. The ethics of evangelism. *Today's Christian Doctor,* Spring 1999:14-16.

Chapter 8

1. VandeCreek L. Patient and family perceptions of hospital chaplains. *Hospital and Health Services Administration* 1991; 36(3):455-467.

2. Fisher M. How do members of an interprofessional clinical team adjust to hospice care? *Palliative Medicine* 1996; 10(4):319-328.

3. Harvey T. Who is the chaplain anyway? Philosophy and integration of hospice chaplaincy. *American Journal of Hospital Palliative Care* 1996; 13(5):41-43.

4. VandeCreek L. Collaboration between nurses and chaplains for spiritual caregiving. *Seminars in Oncology Nursing* 1997; 13(4):279-280.

5. Kaldjian LC, Jekel JF, Friedland G. End-of-life decisions in HIV-positive patients: The role of spiritual beliefs. *AIDS* 1998; 12(1):103-107.

6. Driscoll F. The new congregation: Reflections by an AIDS hospice chaplain. *Journal of Palliative Care* 1995; 11(2):61-63.

7. Puchalski CM. Medical schools teach compassion through taking a spiritual history. *Spirituality and Medical Connection* 1999; 3(1):1.

8. McSherry E, Kratz D, Nelson WA. Pastoral care departments: More necessary in the DRG era? *Health Care Management Review* 1986; 11(1):47-59.

9. Koenig HG. *The healing power of faith.* New York: Simon and Schuster, 1999; 240-247.

10. Field BE, Devich LE, Carlson RW. Impact of a comprehensive supportive care team on management of hopelessly ill patients with multiple organ failure. *Chest* 1989; 96(2):353-356.

Chapter 9

1. George H. Gallup International Institute. Spiritual beliefs and the dying process: A report on a national survey. The Nathan Cummings Foundation and Fetzer Institute, October 1997.

2. Kaldjian LC, Jekel JF, Friedland G. End-of-life decisions in HIV-positive patients: The role of spiritual beliefs. *AIDS* 1998; 12 (1): 103-107.

3. Roberts JA, Brown D, Elkins T, Larson DB. Factors influencing views of patients with gynecologic cancer about end-of-life decisions. *American Journal of Obstetrics and Gynecology* 1997; 176 (1P+1): 166-172.

4. Mickley JR, Soeken, K, Belcher, A. Spiritual well-being, religiousness and hope among women with breast cancer. *Journal of Nursing Scholarship* 1992; 24(4):267-272.

5. Gibbs HW, Achterberg-Lawlis J. Spiritual values and death anxiety: Implications for counseling with terminal cancer patients. *Journal of Counseling Psychology* 1970; 25(6): 563-569.

6. Ringdal GI. Religiosity, quality of life and survival in cancer patients. *Social Indicators Research,* 1996; 38(2):193-211.

7. Yates JW, Chalmer BJ, James P, Follansee M., McKegney FP. Religion in patients with advanced cancer. *Medical and Pediatric Oncology,* 1981; 9(2):121-128.

8. Kaczorowski JM. Spiritual well-being and anxiety in adults diagnosed with cancer. *The Hospice Journal,* 1989; 5(3/4): 105-116.

9. Ellison CW. Spiritual well-being: Conceptualization and measurement. *Journal of Psychology and Theology,* 1983; 11(4): 330-340.

10. King DE, Mansfield C. Do our patients believe in miracles? Presented at the 15th WONCA World Conference, Dublin, Ireland, June 17, 1998.

Chapter 10

1. Pressman P, Lyons JS, Larson DB, Strain JJ. Religious belief, depression, and ambulation status in elderly women with broken hips. *American Journal of Psychiatry* 1990; 147(6):758-760.

2. Harris RC, Dew MA, Lee A, Amaya M, Buches L, Reetz D, Coleman G. The role of religion in heart-transplant recipients' long-term health and well-being. *Journal of Religion and Health* 1995; 34(1):17-32.

3. Conway K. Coping with the stress of medical problems among black and white elderly. *International Journal of Aging and Human Development* 1985-86; 21(1):39-48.

4. King DE, Bushwick B. Beliefs and attitudes of hospital in-patients about faith healing and prayer. *Journal of Family Practice* 1994; 39(4):349-352.

5. Maugans TA, Wadland WC. Religion and family medicine: A survey of physicians and patients. *Journal of Family Practice* 1996; 32(2):210-213.

6. Saudia TL, Kinney MR, Brown KC, Young-Ward L. Health locus of control and helpfulness of prayer. *Heart and Lung* 1991; 20(1):60-65.

7. Florell JL. Crisis-intervention in orthopedic surgery: Empirical evidence of the effectiveness of a chaplain working with surgery patients. *Bulletin of the Professional Hosptial Association* 1973; 37(2):29-36.

8. Oxman TE, Freeman DH, Manheimer ED. Lack of social participation or religious strength and comfort as risk factors for death after cardiac surgery in the elderly. *Psychosomatic Medicine* 1995; 57(1):5-15.

Chapter 11

1. Waldfogel S. Spirituality in medicine. *Primary Care* 1997; 24(4):963-976.

2. Magaletta PR, Ducko PN, Staten SC. Prayer in office practice: On the threshold of integration. *Journal of Family Practice* 1997; 44(3):254-256.

3. Maugans TA. The SPIRITual History. *Archives of Family Medicine* 1996; 5:11-16

4. King DE, Bushwick B. Beliefs and attitudes of hospital inpatients about faith healing and prayer. *Journal of Family Practice* 1994; 39(4):249-352.

5. Matthews DA. Religion and spirituality in primary care. *Mind/Body Medicine* 1997; 2(1):9-19.

6. Lijoi AF. Integrating faith and illness into practice. *Journal of Family Practice 1997*; 45(1):15.

7. Levin JS, Larson DB, Puchalski CM. Religion and spirituality in medicine: Research and education. *Journal of the American Medical Association* 1997; 278(9): 792-793.

8. Puchalski CM, Larson DB. Developing curricula in spirituality and medicine. *Academic Medicine* 1998; 73(9):970-974.

9. Darnard D, Dayringer R, Cassel CK. Toward a person-centered medicine: Religious studies in the medical curriculum. *Academic Medicine* 1995; 70(9): 806-813.

10. Waldfogel S. Wolpe PR, Schmuely Y. *Religious training and religiosity in psychiatry residency programs.* New York: Academic Psychiatry, 1998.

11. Silverman HD. Creating a spirituality curriculum for family practice residents. *Alternative Therapies* 1997; 3(6):54-61.

Index

Page numbers followed by the letter "f" indicate figures; those followed by the letter "t" indicate tables.

AA (Alcoholics Anonymous), 8
Abortion, views on
Catholicism, 16-17
Church of Christ/Protestantism,
17-18
health professionals, 46
Islam, 18
Jehovah's Witnesses, 19
Judaism, 18
Society of Friends (Quakers), 19
Acquired immunodeficiency
syndrome (AIDS), 8, 82. *See
also* HIV-positive patients
Adultery, Church of Christ/Protestant
view on, 17-18
Advocacy, role of chaplains in, 78
African Americans, and religious
commitment, 15
Afterlife, belief in, 90-91
Age, and religious commitment, 16
AIDS (acquired immunodeficiency
syndrome), 8, 82. *See also*
HIV-positive patients
Alcohol use, religious restriction
on, 33
Alcoholics Anonymous (AA), 8
American Association of Medical
Colleges (AAMC), 104
American Psychiatric Association,
46
Anxiety. *See also* Depression;
Mental health
about dying, 86t-87t
in the elderly, 7
in surgical patients, 95-96

Artificial insemination, Catholic
view on, 17
Association of Professional
Chaplains (APC), 73, 75f
Autonomy of patients, 65, 69
Autopsies, views on
Church of Christ/Protestantism, 18
Judaism, 18

Baptists, 14, 15, 71
Biomedical model, 3
Biopsychosocial model, 1-11
Biopsychospiritual model, 6-8
Blacks, religious affiliations of, 15
Blood pressure, effect of religious
involvement on, 5-6, 35
Blood transfusions, views on
Catholicism, 17
Church of Christ/Protestantism, 18
Islam, 18
Jehovah's Witnesses, 19
Breast cancer, patients' responses
to, 4, 89

Cancer, 4, 89
Catholicism, health beliefs of, 17
Center for the Study of
Religion/Spirituality and
Health (Duke University), 31
Chaplains
board certification of, 75
collaboration with physicians,
80-82

Chaplains *(continued)*
    education and training, 73-76,
        77f-78f
    ethics of referral to, 66-68
    impact on patient health, 46, 82-84
    and pastoral services, 73-84
    referral to, 42
    role of, 76-80
Christian Medical and Dental
        Society, 46
Church of Christ, health beliefs
        of, 17-18
Church of Jesus Christ of Latter-Day
        Saints, 15
Circumcision, views on
    Islam, 18
    Jehovah's Witnesses, 19
    Judaism, 18
Clergy, collaboration with
        psychiatrists, 45-46. *See also*
        Chaplains
Clinical ministry program (Loma
        Linda University), 75, 76f,
        77f-78f
Clinical pastoral education, 75-76
Clinical Pastoral Education program
        (UC Davis Health System),
        74f
Clinical practice, integrating
        spirituality into, 99-105
Cognitive-behavior therapy, with
        religious content, 37
Confidentiality, patient, 65-66
Contraception, views on
    Catholicism, 16-17
    Church of Christ/Protestantism, 18
    Islam, 18
    Jehovah's Witnesses, 19
    Judaism, 18
    Society of Friends (Quakers), 19
Coping mechanism
    religion as, 7, 33
    spirituality as, 7, 52, 88-90
Coronary artery disease (CAD),
        and Type A behavior pattern, 3

Counseling, spiritual, 101-102
Crisis counseling, 76
Cults, religious, 32

Death
    anxiety about, 86t-87t, 91
    fear of, 42, 88-89, 91
Demographics, and religious beliefs,
        15-16
Depression, 7, 36-37, 46, 84. *See
        also* Anxiety; Mental health
Diagnosis, presence of chaplain
        during, 80-82
Doctor-patient relationship,
        and biopsychosocial model, 3
Dualism, 3
Dying patients, spirituality
        and, 85-92

Education
    of chaplains, 73-76, 77f-78f
    integrating spirituality into, 10,
        103-105
    in psychiatry programs, 45
Elderly, anxiety and depression in, 7
Ellison Spiritual Well-Being Scale,
        41-42, 89
End-of-life decisions. *See also*
        Death; Terminal illness
    and belief in healing miracles,
        90-91
    role of spirituality in, 86-88
Ethics
    of involvement in patients'
        spirituality, 63-71
    of prayer with patients, 68-69
    of referral to chaplains, 66-68
    of spiritual inquiry, 64-66
Euthanasia, views on
    Catholicism, 17
    Church of Christ/Protestantism,
        17-18
    Islam, 18

Euthanasia, views on *(continued)*
    Jehovah's Witnesses, 19
    Judaism, 18
    Society of Friends (Quakers), 19
Extrinsic religious influence, 8
Extrinsic spirituality, 22

Faith, 24, 59
FICA spiritual assessment tool,
    58-61

Gender, and religious beliefs, 15-16
Geography
    and faith communities, 60
    and religious preferences, 14-15
    and spiritual beliefs of health
        professionals, 40
Ghost, 91
God's will, as factor in healing, 50
Grief counseling, 76
Guilt, 86, 91

Harvard Medical School, 104
Health
    mental, 5, 36, 45-46
    physical, 5-6, 7, 35-36, 82-84
    and religion, reasons to study,
        32-34
    and spirituality, 24-26
Health beliefs of selected religious
        groups, 16-19
Health habits, effect of religious
        affiliation on, 33
Health professionals
    spiritual education of, 103-105
    spirituality of, 39-48
Heaven's Gate, 32
High blood pressure, effect of
        religious involvement on,
        5-6, 35
Hispanics, religious affiliations
    of, 15

HIV-positive patients, 86, 88. *See
    also* AIDS (acquired
        immunodeficiency syndrome)
Holy days, Jewish observance of, 18
Homosexual acts, health
        professionals' views on, 46
Hospital chaplains, 75. *See also*
        Chaplains
Hospitalization
    length of stay, 46, 84, 96
    and spiritual concerns of patients,
        22, 50, 52, 54
Hypertension, effect of religious
        involvement on, 5-6, 35

Illness
    spirituality during, 22-24
    viewed as punishment, 5, 31, 86
Immune function
    effects of religion on, 6, 35-36
    suppression of, 4
In vitro fertilization, Catholic view
    on, 16-17
Inpatients, spiritual concerns of, 52
INSPIRIT Index of Core Spiritual
    Experiences, 9-10, 25-26
Integration gap, 41-43
Intensive care, 55, 84
Interleukin-6 (IL-6) levels, effect of
    religious attendance on, 6, 36
Intrinsic religiousness, 8, 36
Intrinsic spirituality, 22
Islam, health beliefs of, 18

Jehovah's Witnesses, health beliefs
    of, 19
Jonestown, 32
Judaism, health beliefs of, 18

Kasl's Religious Index, 58, 59t, 60

Last rites, 82
Latinos, religious beliefs of, 15

Life satisfaction, 5
Living will, 86
Loma Linda University clinical
    ministry program, 75, 76f,
    77f-78f
Love, Medicine, and Miracles
    (Siegel), 93-94
Lutherans, 14

Mania, 46
Marriage and family therapists,
    religious beliefs of, 39-40
Medical ethics, 63
Medical schools, awareness
    of spiritual issues in, 10
Medication
  pain, 46, 67, 95, 96
  psychotropic, 46
Meditation, and spirituality, 29
Men, religious beliefs of, 15-16
Mental health, 5, 36, 45-46. *See also*
    Anxiety; Depression;
    Physical health
MERIT patient assessment tool, 61
Miracles, 50, 90-91
Mormons, 14, 15
Mortality, effect of religious
    involvement on, 4-5, 34-35
Myocardial infarction, and Type A
    behavior pattern, 3

Neonatal intensive care unit (NICU)
    admissions, and religiously
    affiliated patients, 7-8
Nurses, religious involvement of, 40

Obstetric patients, influence of
    spirituality on, 7-8
Ordination, of chaplains, 75
Outpatients, spiritual concerns of, 52

Pain, effect of religion on, 89, 95-96
Pain medication, reduced need for,
    46, 67, 95, 96
Pastoral services
  and chaplains, 73-84
  impact on patient health, 82-84
Patients
  addressing spiritual concerns
    of, 95-96
  advocacy, 78
  assessing spirituality of, 49-62
  autonomy of, 65, 69
  confidentiality of, 65-66
  desire for addressing spiritual
    issues, 9, 22-24, 50-52
  dying, 85-92
  HIV-positive, 86, 88
  obstetric, 7-8
  privacy of, 65-66, 69
  psychiatric, 50-52
  and religion, 13-20
  satisfaction of, 45
  social and behavioral context
    of, 32-33
  and spirituality, 21-29
  surgical, 93-98
  variation in health beliefs, 33
Physical health, 5-6, 7, 35-36, 82-84.
    See also Mental health
Physicians, religious beliefs
    of, 40-41, 47
Prayer
  ethics of, with patients, 68-69
  influence on biological health, 8
  physicians' use of, 42, 101
  and spirituality, 26-28
  and surgery, 94-95
  to treat alcoholism, 46
  to treat grief, 46
Premarital sex, health professionals'
    views on, 46
Privacy, of patients, 65-66, 69
Protestantism, health beliefs
    of, 17-18
Psychiatric patients, 50-52

Psychiatrists
  religious beliefs of, 41
  views on religion and health,
    45-46
Psychiatry programs, religious
  training in, 45
Psychologists, religious beliefs of, 41
Psychotropic medications, 46
Punishment, illness viewed as, 5, 31,
  86

Quakers (Society of Friends), health
  beliefs of, 19
Quality of care, effect of religion
  on, 46-47

Race, and religious beliefs, 15
Rational-emotive therapy, with
  religious content, 37
Reductionism, 3
Regional religious differences,
  14-15, 40, 60
Religion. *See also* Spirituality
  as coping mechanism, 7, 33, 52,
    88-90
  effect on treatment
    recommendations, 46
  and health, reasons to study, 32-34
  and mortality, 4-5, 34-35
  physiologic effects of, 35-36
  promoting, for better health, 34
  regional differences, 14-15, 40, 60
  in United States, 13-20
  viewed as harmful to health,
    31-32, 45-46
  vs. spirituality, 21
Religious cults, 32
Resuscitation status, and religious
  beliefs, 55, 86, 88
Roman Catholics, 14, 17

Schizophrenia, 46
Seizure disorder, 82

Siegel, Bernie, 93-94
Social support, from religious
  affiliations, 32-33
Society of Friends (Quakers), health
  beliefs of, 19
Spectrum of involvement, 100-103
SPIRIT, 56, 57t
Spiritual assessment instrument
  (INSPIRIT), 9-10, 25-26
"Spiritual distress," as official
  nursing diagnosis, 40
Spiritual healing, 24
SPIRITual history, 26
Spiritual history, 49-62
  and biopsychospiritual model, 6
  how to take, 56-58
  reasons for taking, 10, 49-53,
    100-101
  sample questions, 57t
  when to take, 54-56
Spiritual inquiry
  and confidentiality, 65-66
  as invasion of privacy, 65-66
  objections to, 64-65
  to obtain important medical
    information, 64-65
  and patient autonomy, 65
  rights and responsibilities, 65
Spirituality. *See also* Religion
  assessing, 49-62
  as coping mechanism, 7, 33, 52,
    88-90
  definition of, 21
  in dying patients, 85-92
  in end-of-life decisions, 86-88
  ethics of involvement in, 63-71
  extrinsic, 22
  and health, 24-26
    reasons to study, 32-34
  of health professionals, 39-48
  how to assess, 56-61
  during illness, 22-24
  integrating into clinical practice,
    9-10, 99-105
  intrinsic, 22

Spirituality *(continued)*
  and meditation, 29
  and mental health, 5
  negative effects on health, 31-32
  objections to inquiring about,
      64-65
  and patients, 21-29
  and physical health, 5-6
  positive effects on health, 31
  and prayer, 26-28
  reasons for assessing, 49-53
  in surgical patients, 93-98
  vs. religion, 21
  when to assess, 54-56
"Spirituality and Healing in
      Medicine" (course), 104-105
Spirituality gap, 43-47
Sterilization, views on
  Catholicism, 17
  Islam, 18
Substance use, effect of religion
      on, 5
Suicidal ideation, 5

Surgery, 55, 93-98
Surgical patients, spirituality and, 9,
      50-52, 67, 93-98

Terminal illness, 55, 85-92
Therapists, religious beliefs of, 39-40
Therapy, with religious content, 37
Tobacco use, religious restriction
      on, 33
Training. *See* Education
Twelve-step program, 8
Type A behavior pattern, and
      biopsychosocial model, 3

UC Davis Health System Clinical
      Pastoral Education program,
      74f

What Dreams May Come, 91
Whites, religious beliefs of, 15
Women, religious beliefs of, 15-16

Order Your Own Copy of
This Important Book for Your Personal Library!

FAITH, SPIRITUALITY, AND MEDICINE
Toward the Making of the Healing Practitioner

_____ in hardbound at $49.95 (ISBN: 0-7890-0724-X)

_____ in softbound at $15.95 (ISBN: 0-7890-1115-8)

COST OF BOOKS_____

OUTSIDE USA/CANADA/
MEXICO: ADD 20%_____

POSTAGE & HANDLING_____
(US: $4.00 for first book & $1.50
for each additional book
Outside US: $5.00 for first book
& $2.00 for each additional book)

SUBTOTAL_____

IN CANADA: ADD 7% GST_____

STATE TAX_____
(NY, OH & MN residents, please
add appropriate local sales tax)

FINAL TOTAL_____
(If paying in Canadian funds,
convert using the current
exchange rate. UNESCO
coupons welcome.)

☐ **BILL ME LATER:** ($5 service charge will be added)
(Bill-me option is good on US/Canada/Mexico orders only;
not good to jobbers, wholesalers, or subscription agencies.)

☐ Check here if billing address is different from
shipping address and attach purchase order and
billing address information.

Signature _____

☐ **PAYMENT ENCLOSED: $** _____

☐ **PLEASE CHARGE TO MY CREDIT CARD.**

☐ Visa   ☐ MasterCard   ☐ AmEx   ☐ Discover
☐ Diner's Club   ☐ Eurocard   ☐ JCB

Account # _____

Exp. Date _____

Signature _____

Prices in US dollars and subject to change without notice.

NAME _____

INSTITUTION _____

ADDRESS _____

CITY _____

STATE/ZIP _____

COUNTRY _____ COUNTY (NY residents only) _____

TEL _____ FAX _____

E-MAIL_____

May we use your e-mail address for confirmations and other types of information? ☐ Yes   ☐ No
We appreciate receiving your e-mail address and fax number. Haworth would like to e-mail or fax special
discount offers to you, as a preferred customer. **We will never share, rent, or exchange your e-mail
address or fax number.** We regard such actions as an invasion of your privacy.

Order From Your Local Bookstore or Directly From
The Haworth Press, Inc.

10 Alice Street, Binghamton, New York 13904-1580 • USA
TELEPHONE: 1-800-HAWORTH (1-800-429-6784) / Outside US/Canada: (607) 722-5857
FAX: 1-800-895-0582 / Outside US/Canada: (607) 772-6362
E-mail: getinfo@haworthpressinc.com
PLEASE PHOTOCOPY THIS FORM FOR YOUR PERSONAL USE.
www.HaworthPress.com

BOF00